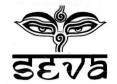

SEVA

The Art of Henna

The Ultimate Body Art Book

Pamela Nichols

HEALTHY PLANET PRODUCTS
Petaluma, CA

Art direction, makeup, hair styling,
and photo styling by Pamela Nichols

Editor: Grace Brumett

Book & Cover design:
Leslie Waltzer
Crowfoot Design Group

Permissions appear on p. 127.
Photography credits and Acknowl-
edgements appear on p. 128.

Healthy Planet Products
Petaluma, CA
1-800-424-4422
www.healthyplanet.com

Distributed to the Book Trade
by Celestial Arts Publishing,
a division of Ten Speed Press

ISBN 0-91686-013-2

Printed in Hong Kong
10 9 8 7 6 5 4 3

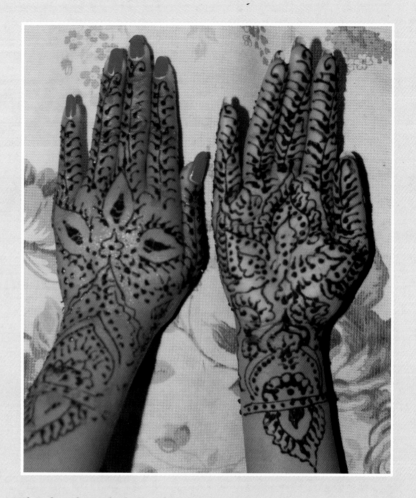

*This book is dedicated to my parents who gave me birth,
to my three beautiful daughters who will always be my muse,
to David Hinds who opened the floodgates of love,
and to the source of all life.*

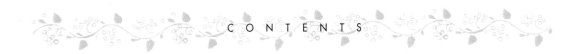

CONTENTS

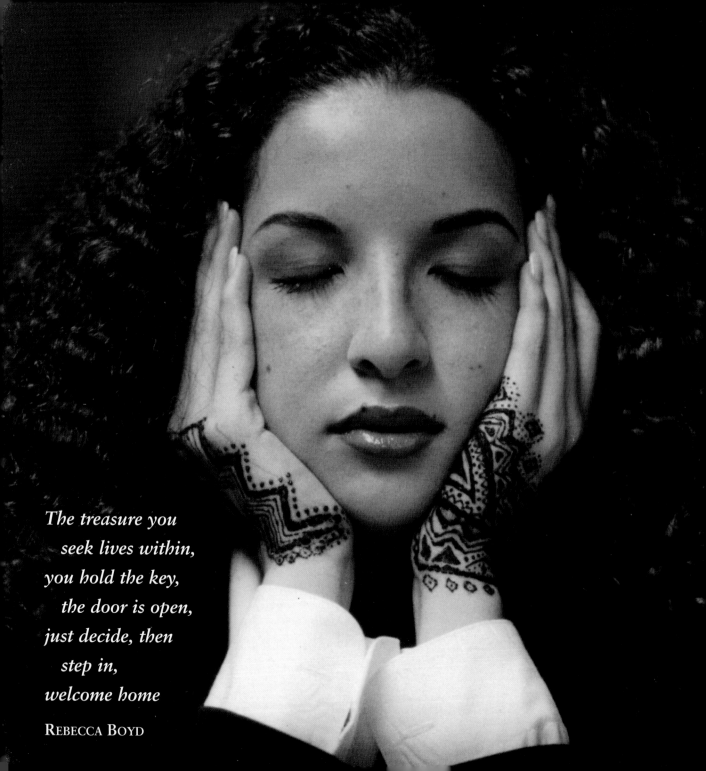

The treasure you
seek lives within,
you hold the key,
the door is open,
just decide, then
step in,
welcome home

REBECCA BOYD

It begins with a story, of course, because henna is about story—personal story. Several years ago, I went on a simple outing with my daughter. Little did I know this journey to a remote town on the beautiful California coast would take me back 5,000 years and link me to an ancient women's art form. Little did I know this invitation to receive a henna design from visiting Pakistani women would become a voyage of my heart. Little did I know I was about to embark on a ritual of love and remembrance that has spanned cultures and generations; a ritual that would nurture and inspire me. I was about to participate in a ritual both sensual and spiritual that is as relevant and alive today at the end of the twentieth century as it has always been.

It began, as all journeys of mystery do, with spontaneity and naiveté. It was summer. My daughter and I plopped into our old beat up station wagon and started up the foggy California coast, delighted to spend time with one another away from life's distractions. I was intrigued with the idea of receiving a henna design. I have always loved decorating my body—and here was an opportunity to adorn myself without the commitment required of a permanent tattoo. At the very least, we would have fun.

When we arrived, several women ushered us into an exquisite room of incense and soft light where we were served Pakistani delicacies and serenaded by musicians from the Far East. It was as though we'd been transported to another time and place. Henna has been used since the time of ancient Egypt and the earliest human cultures. As an American living in such a recently established culture, I've always been fascinated by traditions and rituals that have been passed down through the ages in more ancient societies. In awe, my daughter and I began to understand the significance of henna as an ancient art form.

Hundreds of henna designs were spread before us, and we were asked to choose the one we wanted. After several hours pondering over the right design, as we lounged on beautifully embroidered pillows from an Indian bazaar, my daughter and I began to feel ourselves being transformed. The smolder-eyed women began calmly and quietly drawing on our skin, so warmly and intimately. We reclaimed our ancestry. We were immediately sisters. We became goddesses, feeling with each stroke on our skin a growing sense of beauty, power, strength and mystery. As the designs were painted on our bodies, we were transported magically into other realms. Through the art on our skin we were participating in something primitive and profoundly communal. This art form lends us the time necessary to share stories, laughter and intimacy with one another, time that is so rare in our fast-paced lives. Our imaginations soared with fantasies of desert tribes, mountain shangri-las and mermaids. I understood in my body the value of henna artistry as a ritual at weddings, births and deaths. Henna demands time just to be with one another.

We drove home that starry night over a curvy mountain road through the redwood forest, completely satisfied, nurtured and connected. How did this happen? We laughed in total delight. My daughter's tummy was completely covered with beautiful swirls and flowers and leaves. On my neck and shoulders was an intricate necklace drawn so carefully that it surely looked as if a handsome prince had placed it on me. I felt so comfortable with my body decorated in this way. It was as though henna had evoked a very real and ancient memory that ran deeper than my conscious self.

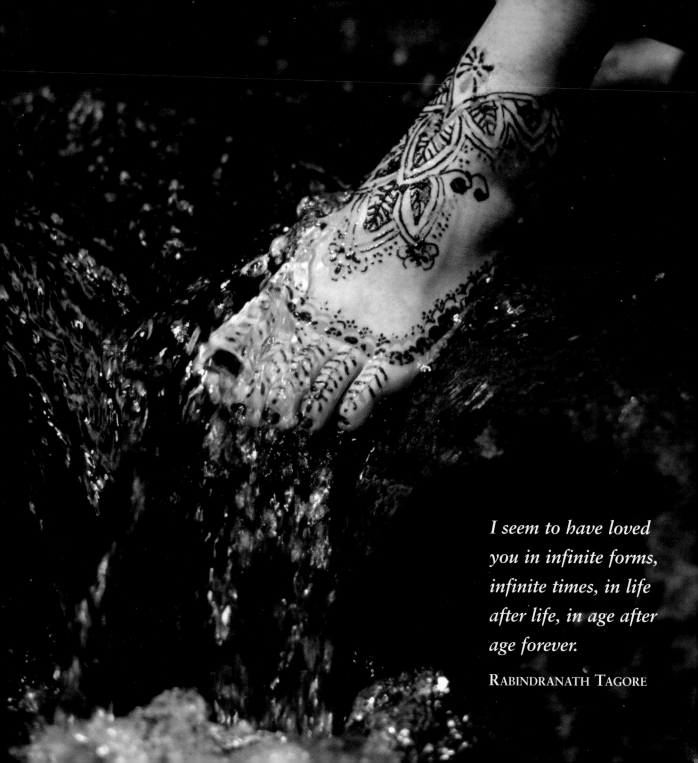

I seem to have loved you in infinite forms, infinite times, in life after life, in age after age forever.

RABINDRANATH TAGORE

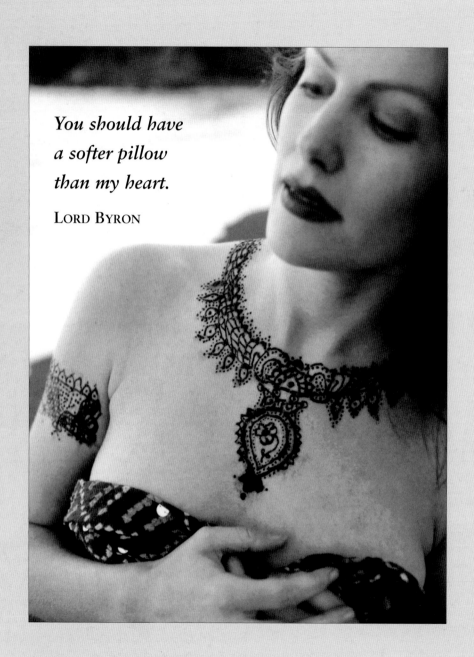

*You should have
a softer pillow
than my heart.*

LORD BYRON

I noticed in the following days how the design seemed to awaken in me and others a very primitive response. This experience of connection continued as I wore my hennaed neckline. What a beautiful experience! I understood how important henna decoration is for our souls, and I recognized how desperately we need these heartfelt experiences in our culture today.

After receiving my henna necklace, I could not stop thinking about henna. I have been a professional makeup artist and hairstylist since 1982, so henna designing became my next natural step. I found several well-known henna artists from India and spent time learning everything I could from them—from the practical details of application to the history and significance of henna in cultures throughout the world.

This ancient art form has traveled through the centuries as an oral tradition passed from hand to hand, woman to woman. Now for the first time in history it is being properly recorded so we all—men and women—can benefit from knowing this rich tradition.

Step forth now and enjoy. Take part in this book. I will guide you on a journey through the world of henna. You will be inspired by artful photographs and discover a collection of designs and stencils from many cultures. You will receive step-by-step henna application instructions. You will read tips and advice useful for beginners and advanced students of henna. You will learn henna's historical roots and traditions. I will tell you little stories of joy-making.

I invite you to begin.

◄ *A henna neckline design inspired from an ancient Indian silver waist belt.*

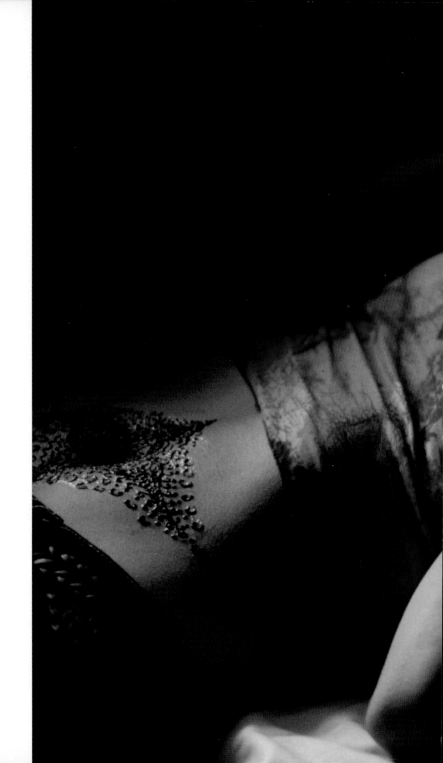

If I hold her hand
She says, "Don't touch!"
If I hold her foot
She says, "Don't touch!"
But when I hold
her waist beads
She pretends not to know.

AFRICAN VILLAGE WEDDING SONG

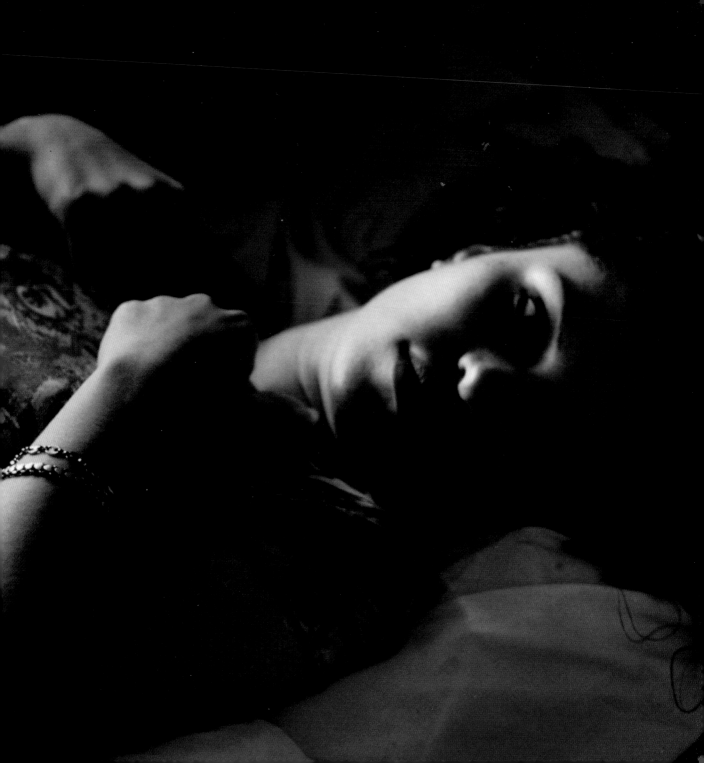

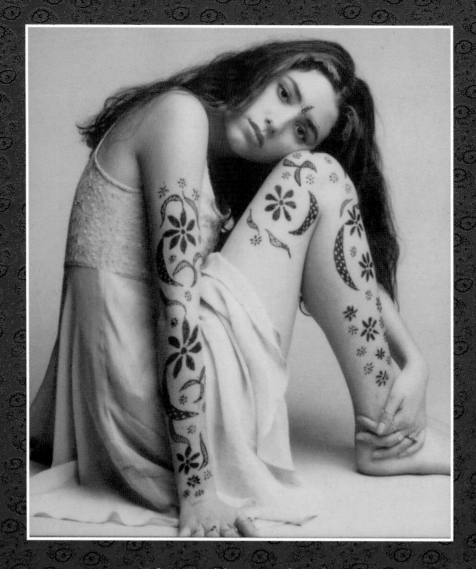

The World is our family.

MAHA UPANISHAD

Since the beginning of time, people all over the world have tattooed or decorated their bodies. Anthropologists have found enough evidence from ruins and artifacts to show that permanent and temporary tattooing have flourished for the last 15,000 years.

Tattoos have been found in the ancient artifacts and records of Crete, Greece, Persia and Arabia. By 2000 B.C. tattoos had appeared in China. Tattoos have been found in the Neolithic period approximately 7000 years ago. People of the Philippines, South Sea Islands, Australia, New Zealand and such cultures as the Maya, Aztec, Haida and most indigenous tribes of North America all used temporary body decoration from plant mixtures.

Tattoos have symbolized visions, journeys, battles, love, protection and membership in a certain tribe or clan. Celtic warriors would paint their bodies with blue dye. If they were captured or killed during battle they would be identified by the color of their country. In Britain, the Anglo-Saxon King Harold had his body heavily tattooed. As the story goes, when women recovered his body after the battle of Hastings, they found "Edith" tattooed across his heart. King George V of France, Czar Nicholas II of Russia and King Frederik IX of Denmark all wore tattoos. In Borneo, specific tattoos on a woman's forearm showed that she was a highly skilled weaver, and thus she would be a very marriageable woman. It was also believed that tattoos on both the fingers and wrists of men and women would keep away illness.

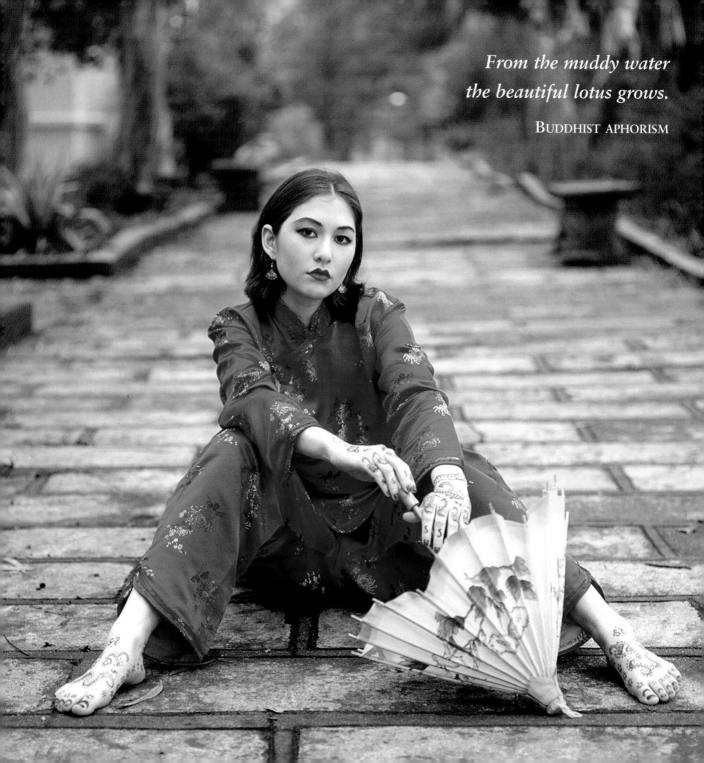

*From the muddy water
the beautiful lotus grows.*

BUDDHIST APHORISM

People from all over the world have always used body markings in the form of piercings or tattoos, whether permanent or temporary. And people have always used plants as their allies—ingesting them, smoking them, applying them to the body in one way or another. Who was the first woman to rub henna leaves on her body and find it beautiful? When did foraging nomads first discover the value of this odd scrubby plant which would ultimately become so instrumental in their lives?

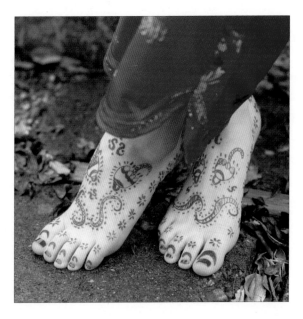

Modern Indian henna design of umbrellas, depicting everyday life.

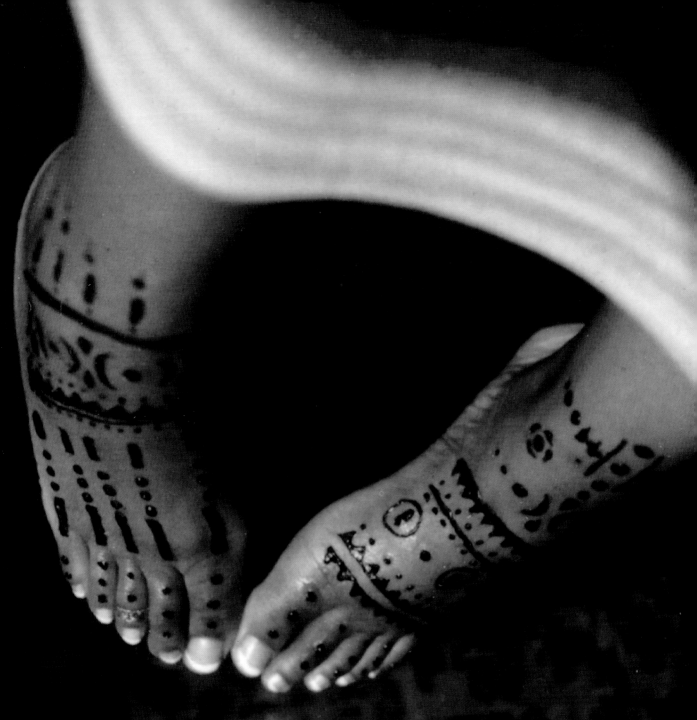

Lovers do not finally meet somewhere, they are in each other all along. JELALUDDIN RUMI

When did henna become a sacred vehicle of transformation and good fortune? When did it first lend itself to human rites of passage, offering protection and beauty? No one knows for sure, but there are many clues.

ASSYRIA

In a fertile valley near the moist banks of the Tigris River in the ancient Empire of Assyria lived a people who believed in good and evil spirits; who believed in magic. They wrote their histories in ink on parchment paper that decayed long ago. Yet fragmentary remains from their culture suggest the henna plant was widely used there. King Ashurbanipal, their last great king, was a dreaded warrior, a patron of the arts, and a handsome gentleman. It is said he took a cosmetic case to war containing henna to color his nails and the palms of his hands. Entering the battlefield, he was immaculately groomed. In the quiet graves at Susa and El-'Ubeid brave warriors lie, their beards, hair and eyebrows are stained with henna.

EGYPT

Evidence of henna use going back 5,000 years can be found in the royal tomb of Ramses II in Egypt. The nails of his shrouded body are painted with henna as are the soles of his feet. His hair is dyed a burnt red henna and his palms are saturated with henna. The shrouds of fabric wrapping his mummified body are dyed with henna as final protection.

◄ *An ancient Egyptian henna design.*

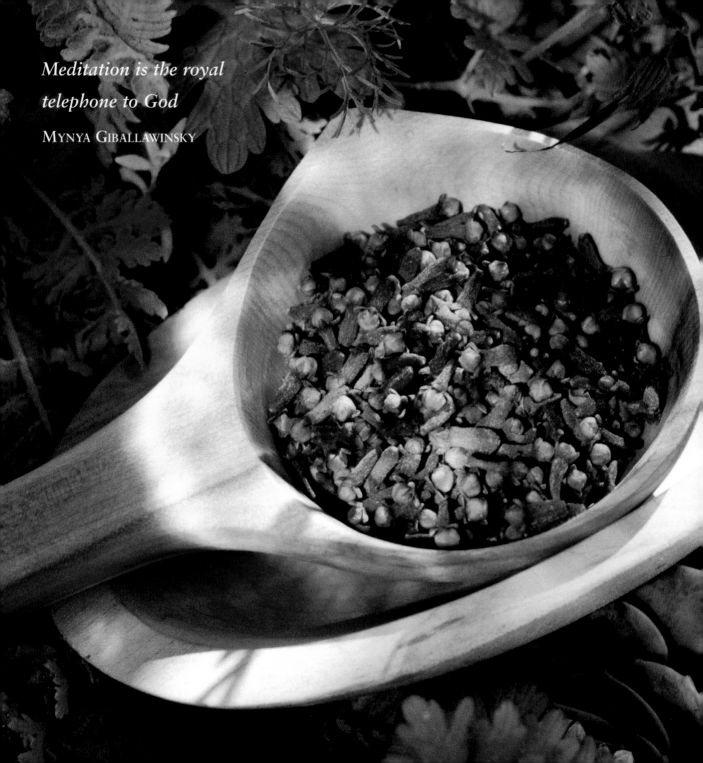

*Meditation is the royal
telephone to God*

MYNYA GIBALLAWINSKY

At sunset, the ancient Egyptians would burn the henna plant as an incense to invoke the spirit of Ra. Ra, the god of the sun, represented all that is born and not yet born. It was believed that when henna was burned in ritual sacrifices, the smoke of the plant rising to the heavens served to rouse Ra. Being pleased, he would then remember to send peace into the lives of the Egyptian people.

Even the Bible mentions the use of henna. When the Hebrew tribes led by Moses fled Egypt, this was written: "My beloved is like a cluster of henna blossoms in the orchard of Engedi." (Song of Solomon 1:14)

During the third and fourth dynasties when the great pyramids were being built, Cleopatra went to extreme lengths to protect and enhance her renowned beauty with henna. She would comb a henna rinse through her long black hair and dip her hands and feet in earthen vessels of henna tea to protect herself from the hot Egyptian sun.

The women of this long ago time would go out and gather henna leaves from the banks of the Nile in baskets. They knew exactly where to find the best plants. They dried the leaves in a dark place then ground them into a fine powder at exactly the right moment. Later still, they mixed this potion with water to make a paste. Using a narrow sliver of wood as an applicator, they placed henna paste on their hands and feet to look as beautiful as possible.

◄ *A ladle filled with whole cloves, a common ingredient in henna paste.*

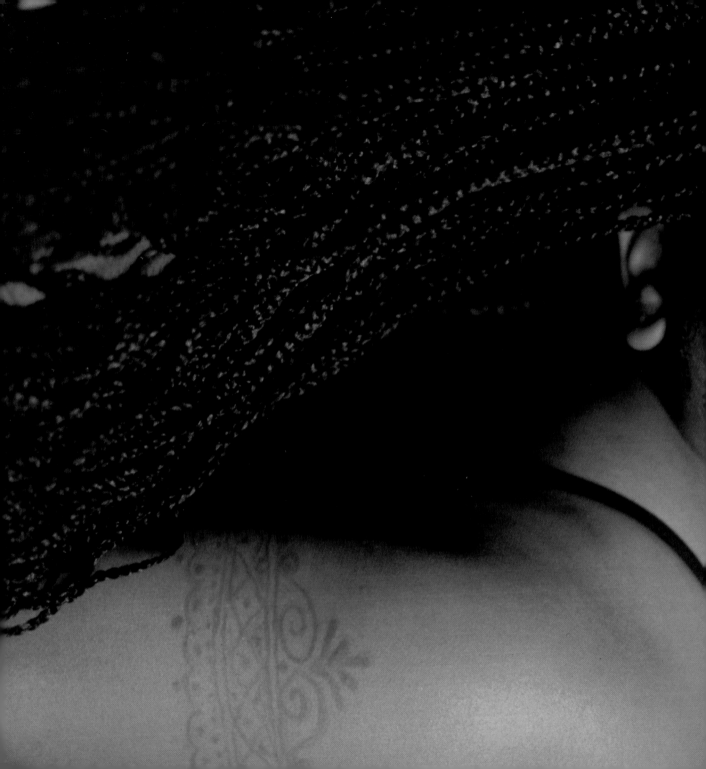

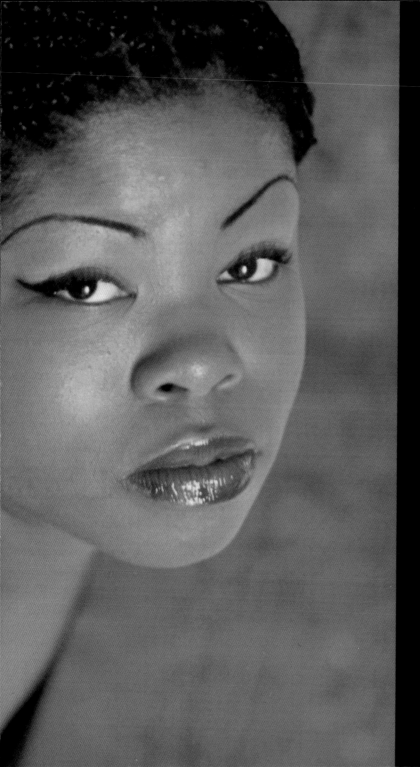

If I *have prophetic powers,
and understand all mysteries
and have all faith so to move
mountains but have not love,
I am nothing.*

I CORINTHIANS 13:2

◄ *A beautiful armband design inspired
by the headdress of a Central Asian bride
from a royal family.*

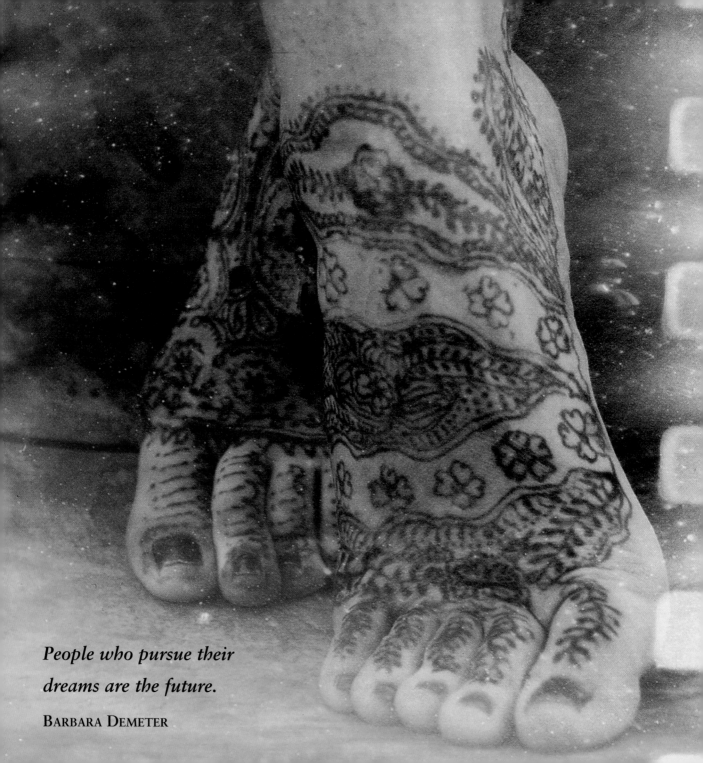

People who pursue their dreams are the future.

BARBARA DEMETER

Time passed and henna, the plant of love, found its way across the Mediterranean to Rome—most fittingly on the hands and feet of Cleopatra, the Egyptian queen of beauty, who had tempestuous love affairs first with Julius Caesar and then Mark Antony. Hers was a tale of great passion and jealousy. She crossed the Mediterranean to marry Julius Caesar. With her to the shores of Rome went baskets of henna—in the arms of her faithful handmaidens. As Cleopatra and Mark Antony fell deeply in love, the henna seeds the beautiful Egyptian queen brought with her were firmly planted in the soil of Rome.

Intrigue and ill will festered between Antony and his rival, Octavian, over this union. Mark Antony and his famed lover returned to Egypt, where word reached Cleopatra that Octavian was coming to kill her beloved Antony. She hurriedly boarded one of her naval ships with sails soaked in perfume, plumes of incense billowing. She set out to sea to warn Antony of the impending danger. She was desperate to save his life. Tragically, the tale ends when the lovers take their own lives. Henna, though, had reached the shores of Rome on the arms of Cleopatra, following her in her passion for two of the greatest Roman leaders of the day.

Morocco

Out of this union between Cleopatra and Mark Antony came an exquisite, delicate girl child, Cleopatra Selene, the darling of the court. Word of her beauty spread along the trade routes across the Atlas and

Rif Mountains of Northern Africa into Morocco, the land of the Berbers. These were herding and farming tribes whose history dates to 3,000 B.C. As they coursed across the barren desert on slow moving camels laden with gold and ivory, they brought back tales of the bewitching charms of this young and nubile beauty. It was rumored that she was living in Rome as a captive. The young scholarly son of King Juba I was also in Rome. He, too, had been taken as a child from his homeland as a spoil of war.

Word soon arrived along the caravan routes that the little Egyptian princess had been given in marriage to the tall, darkly handsome King Juba II. Soon they would cross the sea to reign together in Morocco. And so it was. She became his bride and prepared to leave. With her came her court of women and all her potions, amongst them henna. For, of course, she had always used henna for beauty.

Morocco is a land at once exotic and mysterious. Long narrow streets of the Medina wind endlessly, laced with people in striking robes of brilliant hues. Veiled women walk hand in hand speaking only with their eyes to those they pass. The senses are assaulted by the smells of sweet mint tea and pungent spices. Dark men squat behind baskets on bright colored blankets, flutes in hand, seducing snakes to twist and entrance.

Storytellers on the corner weave tales for days on end, pausing at just the right moment. Wide-eyed listeners beg, "Please go on," and toss coins. The story goes on. In this harsh land one feels the need for protection from the evil spirits. One feels the presence of the *jinni*. These invisible beings from the spirit world demand much attention and appeasement to make dreams come true. One can lose one-self here, as Jimi Hendrix did centuries later.

▸ *A Berber design frequently seen in Morocco.*

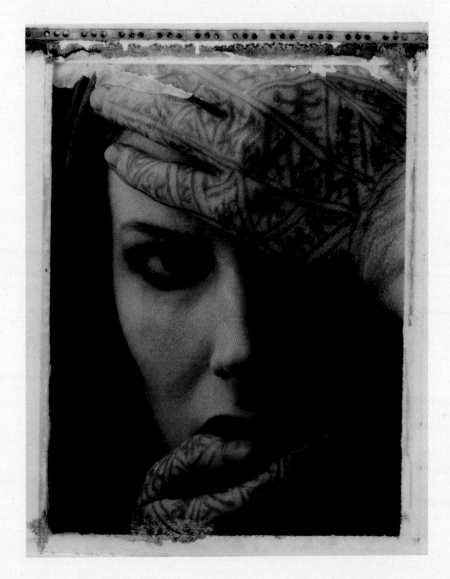

I am woman, mysterious and eternal.

Isabel Allende

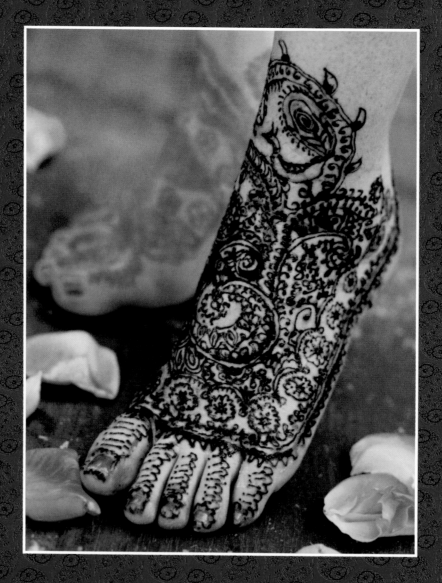

Nothing in life is to be feared, it is only to be understood.

MAHA UPANISHAD

Go back now with me and watch. Cleopatra Selene arrives at this foreign shore. She and her ladies mingle with the women of Morocco. These heavily veiled women have eyes darkened by kohl, which burn like powerful magnets. As with women everywhere, intimacies grow, stories are told, beauty secrets exchanged. The customs between these women interweave.

Cleopatra Selene brought henna to Morocco only to find that it was already there. Cleopatra's daughter was to learn more about the secrets of henna, because in Morroco the use of henna went beyond the purposes of beautification and adornment. Here, henna eroticizes a woman who must live behind veils. Henna parties are called to help a woman who is troubled or when there is a need to contact the spirit world.

A henna party is about to commence. The female seer (*shuwafa*) who acts as a consultant has arrived. She calls in Lalla Malika, the most esteemed *jinni* in Fez, whose favorite henna designs are the most intricate. Lalla Malika loves orange blossom water and incense. "Come with us tonight, Cleopatra Selene," the seer says. "We must grant Lalla Malika her wish or she will cause much trouble."

The women join together to help, as women do everywhere. The henna party is for mature women. Here, out of the public eye and with friends, Cleopatra Selene is safe to contact these highly dangerous spiritual forces. Her problems will be taken seriously with the communal support of her sisters. This event is one of liberation.

◄ *A Rajasthani wedding design for the feet. The foot in the foreground has just been hennaed. On the foot in the background, the process is complete.*

For three days, Cleopatra Selene receives henna decorations on both her hands and feet. Each morning the henna is scraped off with a silver bangle and reapplied to get the darkest stain possible. She is then wrapped in scarves to protect the henna while she sleeps. For three days she must remain almost immobile.

On the third day the henna is baked onto her skin over aromatic coals to darken it even more. The seer, in a trance, is present to examine the wishes of the *jinni*. Harmony must be established. The last day of the henna party arrives. Cleopatra Selene reclines amid her friends and handmaidens, wrapped in gorgeous robes. Incense perfumes the room. It is sunset. The room is aglow.

Cleopatra Selene delicately moves the rising smoke toward her face and breathes in the incense. It is night. The music begins and the women twist sinuously. Their jewelry glitters. They dance around her. The energy becomes more intense. The pulsing rhythm awakens the *jinni* who has now possessed the henna-adorned woman. The *jinni* enters her body. She rises and begins to pulsate slowly. More incense is placed under her.

Suddenly an intense expression crosses her face. She enters the land of the *jinni*. The music gets stronger. All body movements become more frenetic as more women join the trance, writhing and twirling around her. Scarves come untied. Hair swirls. Eyes fill with tears. The presence of the *jinni* is felt. Finally the trance comes to an end. The women collapse on the floor where they are taken care of until they revive. The women of Cleopatra Selene's court go home. They have been initiated.

▸ *Hennaed hands inspired from a 1950's fabric design.*

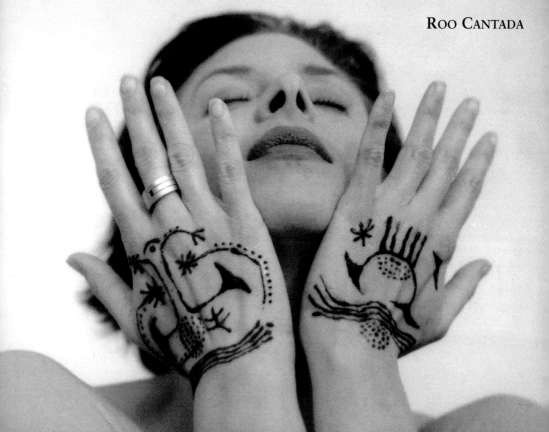

You make me delirious,
spinning high and oblivious,
grinning from ear to ear,
wandering so far . . .

ROO CANTADA

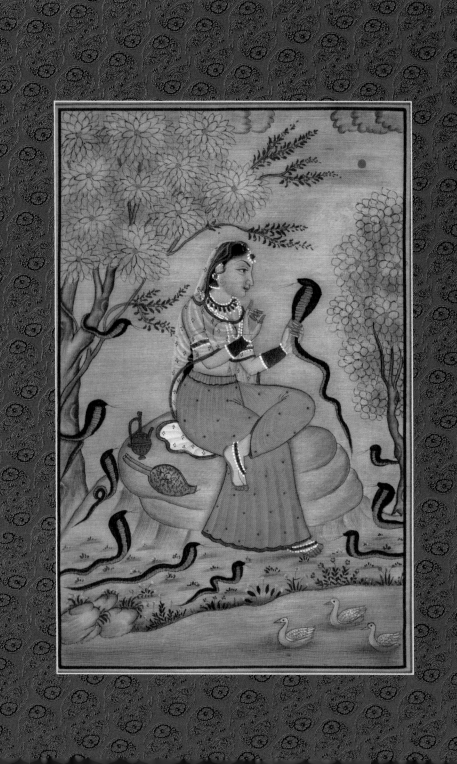

INDIA

No one is certain when henna came to India. Some think henna actually has its roots in India from prehistoric times. From there it may have scattered and dispersed floating onto the shores of Egypt much later. Henna in India is surrounded with much mystery. Unlike Egypt, where the hot dry climate preserves artifacts for centuries, the humid climate of India has destroyed many clues. Also the belief in reincarnation puts no significance on recording details of daily personal or cultural life—so historical records are minimal. So we do not know exactly when henna entered human culture. We know only that it has been present in India for at least 3,000 years as an important part of her history. We also know that almost every festival in India is marked with women decorating their hands with henna.

In India, beautification is only one of henna's uses. Henna is also used as a hair conditioner and served as the very first sun block. The Indian people have always worked hard out in the fields every day exposed to the elements. Henna was applied for centuries to the soles of the feet and palms of the hands for protection against the harsh wind and sun. The people of India also recognized the cooling quality of henna. In the hotter regions they have traditionally applied it to the feet and palms to draw out body heat. Since ancient times, when cooking with strongly aromatic herbs was common, women would put henna on their palms. The delicate scent would cancel the rather powerful pungency of their kitchen spices. Henna has all of these practical uses. Primarily it has been a woman's herb. In the many stages of a woman's life, especially in traditional ceremonies, henna has played an important role.

◄ *An interpretation of an 18th Century Aswari Ragini miniature painting from India showing hennaed hands and feet.*

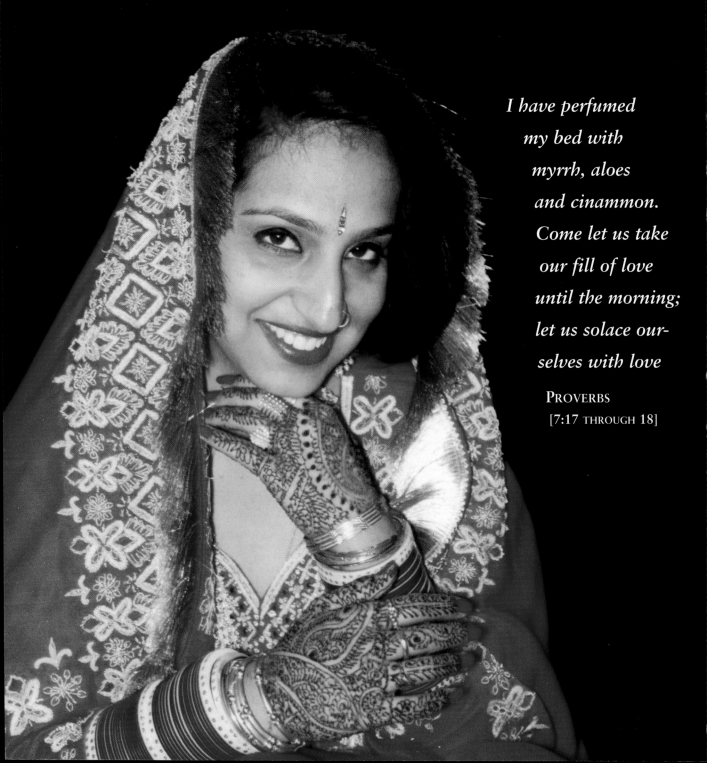

*I have perfumed
my bed with
myrrh, aloes
and cinammon.
Come let us take
our fill of love
until the morning;
let us solace our-
selves with love*

PROVERBS
[7:17 THROUGH 18]

One of the most joyful rites of human passage is the celebration of love through marriage. So, of course, henna is used as part of the wedding ceremony in many cultures and countries. Join me on a romantic tour of wedding ceremonies throughout the world.

INDIA

Traditional Indian women are taught to look forward to their wedding ceremony as the most important ritual in their lives. *The Kama Sutra*, an ancient Indian book of love, offers preparation to girls as they enter the world of adult women. It encourages every young girl to partake in henna designs.

Studying the history of henna, I really wanted to understand these women, living in a culture so different from my own. How did they feel? How could I understand women of eastern cultures, who appear to my western eyes as subservient? I had to discard all my preconceptions to truly understand. So I turned to India's mythology, captured in this beautiful love tale about the gods Rama and Sita. This story depicts how a young bride might see herself.

Rama and Sita were the perfect divine couple. Sita became the perfect goddess wife of Hinduism. One day Rama and Sita were married. God told Rama he must go into the forest for fourteen years. Rama loved Sita and worried it would be too hard for her in the forest. He decided she could not go with him. Sita, in her intense anguished love and devotion, wrote him pages and pages, pouring from

◂ *Henna designs on the hands for a modern Indian wedding.*

her heart. She knew she would die if he left without her. She stated all the reasons why she should go with him. She finally convinced Rama. Together they left. Far out in the wild forest she bore him two children. In giving up worldly life Sita showed her great and pure love and devotion. Through the power of her love, she gained the ear of god. This lent her great power.

This beautiful Indian myth is recited over and over to every young Indian girl from the time she is very young. It reveals an Indian woman's real sense of devotion at the marriage ceremony. She recognizes within herself the goddess aspect of Sita who has the ear of god. In the marriage ceremonies of Hindu India, these vows of love and devotion are recited. Putting henna on her hands as preparation is a symbol of the bride's desire to be in devotional union. She shows her husband her most incredible beauty with the application of henna. Many paintings, weavings and wall carvings show goddesses and women alike hennaed with beautiful designs representing their love. You can see this in the cave paintings of Ajanta and Allora.

Of all the ceremonies in India where henna is used, the wedding ceremony is the most important and powerful rite of passage. Imagine the sense of excitement the young, shy bride and groom must feel as they approach it, aware how their lives will now be forever changed.

The marriage ritual in Northern India is called *vivaha*. This is how it has always been for over 3,000 years:

The bride and groom are separate from one another the entire week prior to the wedding day preparing their bodies. Each part of the ritual serves to purify, beautify and symbolically prepare the couple. The beauty ritual starts with a daily ceremony of "taking up oil." The skin of the bride is carefully rubbed with a mixture of honey and oil mixed with special herbs to tint it red and yellow.

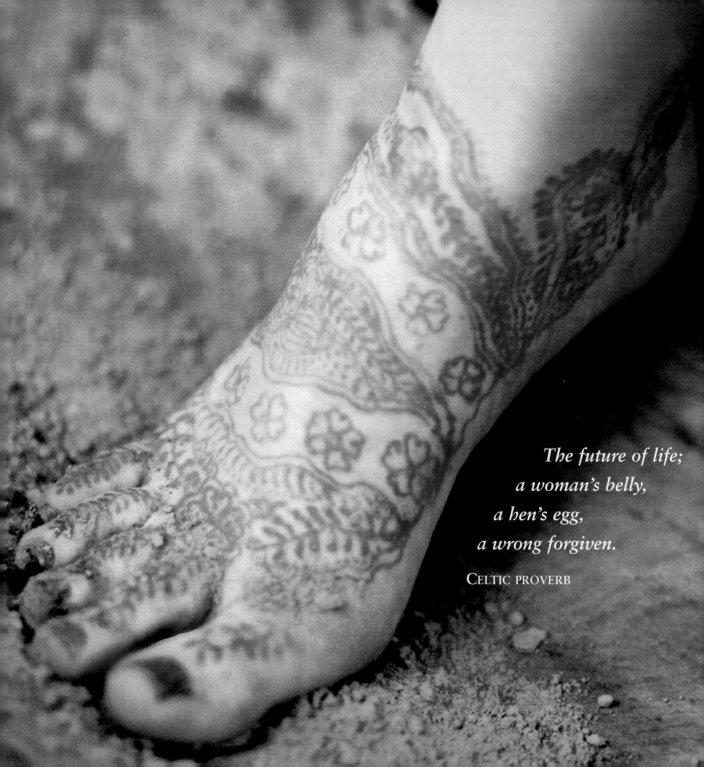

The future of life;
a woman's belly,
a hen's egg,
a wrong forgiven.

CELTIC PROVERB

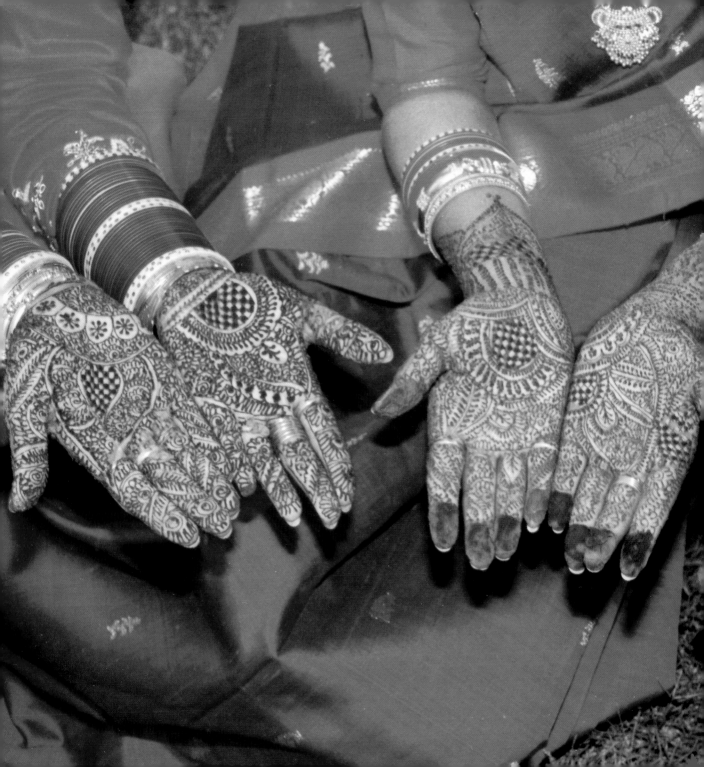

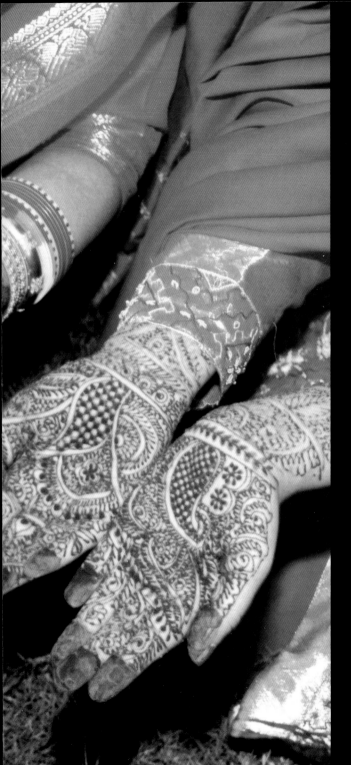

My love, bring to me quickly
the deepest red colored mehndi possible,
and I will tint both of my hands.
When my hands are beautifully decorated,
I will bow at the feet of your mother,
and receive her blessings.
We will then live so happily together.
So my dearest love,
bring the darkest staining mehndi
and for our union
I will decorate my hands.

Rajasthani folk song

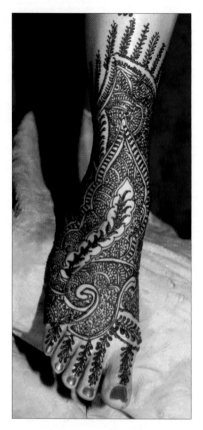

Red is preferred as the color of good luck. After some time this mixture is taken off leaving the skin smooth, tender and pure. A paste of oatmeal flour, butter and turmeric is then applied to remove body hair. It nourishes the skin giving it a sunny glow. Now the skin is properly prepared for a long lasting henna design.

Finally, *mehendi raat*, the Night of Henna has come. Henna paste arrives from the groom's family. The sister-in-law is the one to decorate the hands and feet of the bride. As she painstakingly draws the elaborate and intricate designs, the women sing songs of love and joy.

In the traditional way, the bride's hands are decorated past the wrist and her feet are decorated past the ankles with the most incredible lacy designs called *mehendi*. Both sides of her hands are decorated. This symbolizes that each hand is really two hands. She will be able to give twice as much love to her husband. The bride feels so honored to adorn herself in this way.

It is said that if anyone accidentally touches the wet henna from the bride's hands and feet she will be married very soon. I'm sure there is much touching! Finally the hands and feet of the young bride are wrapped in cotton cloth to protect the designs for the next 6 to 12 hours. She remains passive and receptive to all the loving attention.

Meanwhile, in another place, the groom is also being prepared the day before the wedding. He bathes in milk, honey and mustard oil. His mother, or a female relative, first applies a cream of turmeric, flower essences, beautifully scented oils and ghee to his feet, hands and face. This will wipe away any darkness. Next the tops and bottoms of his hands are adorned with henna as a symbol of his devotion to his wife and to his marriage.

The wedding day finally arrives. Early in the morning the bride washes her hands in wonderfully scented rose water. Her uncle places red colored bangles on her wrists to compliment her beautifully ornate and lacy scrolled hands and feet.

Everyone awaits in great anticipation. "What will she look like?" they wonder.

The bride appears in her brilliant red sari, red bangles on her hands and feet, and henna on her skin. Everyone gasps in delight. The

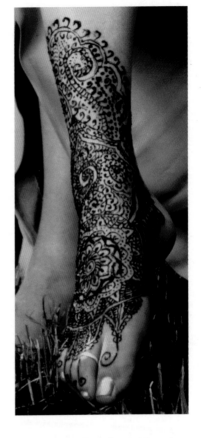

marriage ceremony begins. The sister-in-law places a bowl of henna in the new couple's clasped hands as they go around the sacred fire. They do this simple dance to symbolically transfer the love from the groom's family to the newlyweds. The vows of Rama and Sita are enacted once more.

Seeing this bride in her traditional sari, you think it could well be the year 1,000. Her hands and feet are covered with traditional patterns made of closely networked lines, squares, triangles and diamonds. Although, looking closely at the henna patterns, some might show more modern designs and motifs which combine flower patterns with candies, clothes, animals, birds and insects. Not much has really changed over the centuries. The bride is beautiful and henna adorns her.

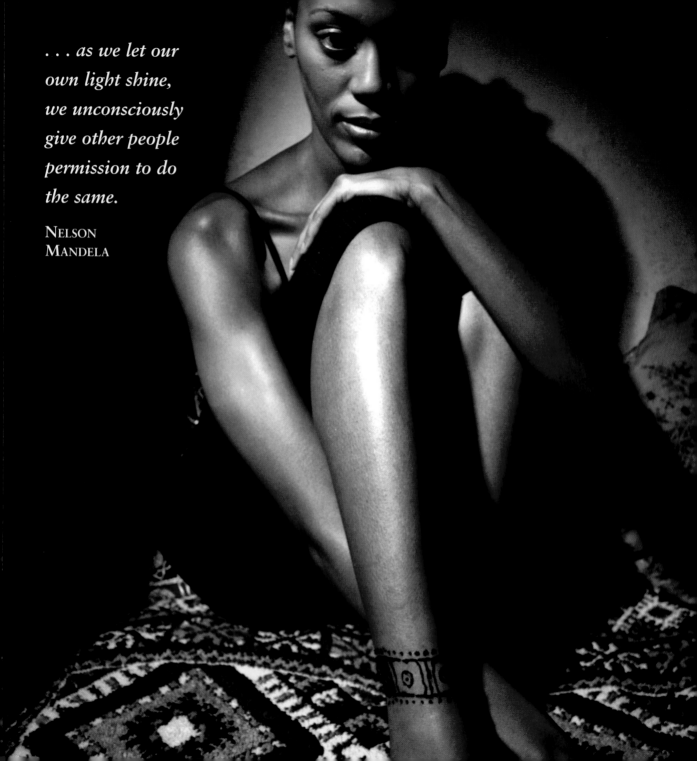

. . . as we let our own light shine, we unconsciously give other people permission to do the same.

NELSON
MANDELA

MUSLIM WEDDING TRADITIONS

Muslim weddings in India have a playful tradition involving henna. Before the wedding the groom's sister and her girlfriends deliver henna to the groom. Then they linger and relentlessly tease him about his new life.

The Muslim bride on her way to the marriage ceremony is carried by her friends so that she can reach above the door. She places her wet hennaed hands on the high wall of her parents' house making a hand print. This gesture symbolizes her farewell to her parents' home as she moves in with her husband's family. It is an occasion for tearful joy.

EGYPT

The modern bride in Egypt finds henna very important in her wedding ceremony. In preparation for her wedding day, she secrets herself away with all her female relatives and bridesmaids. Together there is much feasting and feminine merriment. The women sing songs of love to her. The finest batch of henna is selected and carefully prepared. The women mix it into a fine paste as they sing, chatter and giggle together, and they tell all the stories the young bride needs to hear. Into the hand of the bride the mother places a spoonful of henna. It is a blessing time for all. Each woman sticks a golden coin into the henna on the bride's hand. Remember the old fairy tale where the twelve fairies of the kingdom arrive to bless the princess Sleeping Beauty. Surely they were the wise elder women. This henna, having been blessed by each woman, is scraped into a cup of water and stirred into a fine paste for later. More henna is applied to the bride's hands and feet. They are wrapped in fine linen until morning.

It is a night of dreams for the young virgin bride as she prepares to embark from this night with so much feminine love surrounding her into her future life as a wife. The rest of the wedding party stay with her. They use the remaining henna to adorn the palms of their own hands. Everyone is blessed. This special night is called the "Night of the Henna." It is a tradition that spans the centuries.

MOROCCO

Today in Morocco henna parties are important in the very same way they were in ancient times. Seers are called in. Trances are induced. Women support one another. Henna decorating is considered vital for a girl's transition into womanhood, and so it is very important in the wedding ceremony.

From the time they are very little, girls sit upon earthen steps and practice doing henna on their mothers' hands. All the women come to watch. They give advice on how to produce the best red-orange henna and the nicest designs. Later, at her wedding ceremony, henna will help her transition to womanhood with all its new responsibilities. These are the Berber people and this is their tradition.

A wedding is about to commence. A henna artist (*mu-'allima*) is called upon at this time. She begins the designs on the first of the three-day wedding ceremony. Before the bride begins her designs she will be bathed in aromatic herbs and fragrant oils, to insure her physical and spiritual purity. She must also fast for these three days to further assure her purification. The bride's mother mixes the henna paste from a recipe handed down from woman to woman, generation to generation.

As with any style of fashion, the henna designs differ from one country to another. Within Morocco they differ from village to village. Some designs show a great deal of delicacy. Such a design can begin with one decorated finger or cover the whole hand. The designs have no implicit meaning, since the Islamic religion forbids representational forms taken from the culture or from nature. However, the designs have great power. Composed of very thin lined geometric motifs, they form patterns called "the eye of God." These designs are believed to provide a protective barrier to dispel all evil from the bride—and only a woman who has been married just one time can apply the design.

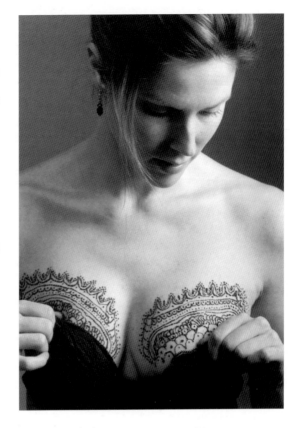

The ceremonies continue. The room is filled with the sweet scent of incense burning on hot coals. Provocative and joyful music fills the room in which the women gather, sipping orange blossom water, singing songs, telling jokes and stories, and advising the new bride on the secrets of married life. The women dance around the bride for the purpose of invoking good spirits, good luck and dispelling all fears. This ritual will ensure the bride the great fortune of having a good marriage. Men can be present only to play music or in service to the bride.

The grooms of Morocco also use henna in the wedding ceremony. The night before the wedding, the groom's house is carefully cleaned and purified with incense, prayers and music. Spells are cast to remove any negative obstacles that might be in the way of a happy, fertile and prosperous marriage.

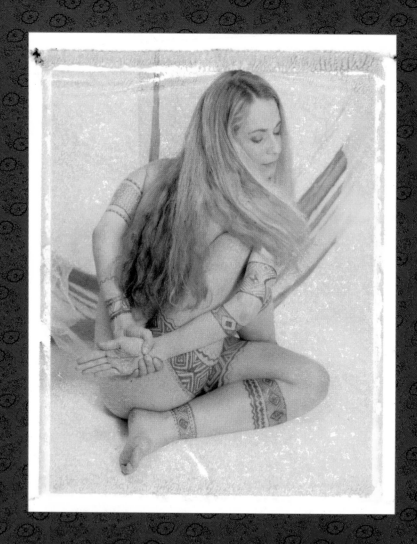

. . . by refrigerator light
her bending body
through a new kimono

STEVE SANFIELD

The night before the wedding, the bride is brought to the groom's house. They partake of a feast with family, friends and neighbors. They celebrate and chase away evil spirits by firing guns in the air. In the wee hours of the next morning, the groom and his male friends gather together and walk through the town accompanied by men playing musical instruments.

When the men finally return to the groom's house in the morning, his mother meets them at the door. She hands them a bowl of henna, an egg (representing fertility), a bottle of water (symbolizing prosperity), and four candles (symbolizing purification). The best man puts henna on his own hands, and one by one he lights the candles, and places them in the henna bowl. The groom's party stands in a circle, and passes the bowl filled with henna around to one another. When each of the men has touched the bowl, the best man drops the henna bowl on the hard tile floor. It breaks open to symbolize the breaking of the hymen.

TUNISIA

Can you smell the hot African desert? It is night and the pots have been boiling for three days now as women prepare delicious stews and puddings for the wedding feast. The nomadic tribe members sit on beautifully woven rugs preparing for the wedding. The bride's friends stir and cook down the sweet syrup that will be spread on her skin to remove her body hair. Her skin must be soft and smooth, ready for her wedding night.

The henna designs to adorn her are primitive tribal motifs. They are geometric and angular, reflecting nomadic life. A pool of ripened henna paste is placed on a flattened small stick and thin lines are slowly dripped upon the bride's skin. They will form patterns to cover the top and the bottom of her hands and feet in preparation for her wedding These designs are symbols of protection and a declaration of eternal love. In delight she thinks of her happy marriage to come and asks the gods to render her fertile.

NIGER

Now move through the desert of North Africa. Feel the breezes sweep across the hot sand, cooling the land, as the nomadic Tuareg tribe settles for the night. We creep closer to the fire. We hear a story. It is a tale of the desert about men who ride proudly on their camels with their faces veiled, showing only their noble and fierce eyes. They move in a slow caravan carrying ostrich feathers, salt, parrots and ivory. Their tents are made of strong, tough leather.

They make camp. The women prepare a dessert of crushed sweet dates in large bowls for everyone to eat. They add water from a gourd. This tribe knows all the secret springs on the vast empty desert. Bathed in the glow of the fire we soon fall asleep.

In the morning thin pancakes are served with sweet mint tea called *atai*. These are the desert traders of long ago. As the sun slinks behind the dunes we hear the sound of drum beats and the rhythm of animal hooves. They blend with high voices singing an almost forgotten melody. The Tuareg men of Niger come home from a long journey crossing the shifting sands of the desert, wearing long blue robes. These Tuareg men are called the *Blue People*. All the robes are dyed indigo. The skin underneath turns blue from the stain. The darker the skin is stained, the wealthier is the man. Before the wedding a man will darken his eyes and brows with ashes before donning his veil. It is a matriarchal society where women own the land and can declare a divorce. It is a society governed by the words found in an old weathered text, "To wander is to be free . . ."

We find a shy groom being prepared. Everywhere these long blue-robed people come in and out of tents. In this desert region of Air-in-Niger, the Tuareg men celebrate their love for their brides-to-be by having henna applied to their hands and feet. They believe this is a symbol of purity and fertility, as well as protection from evil spirits.

The nuptial tent, *ehan*, is made of wooden poles laced together and covered with beautiful, hand-woven, brightly colored blankets. Women have constructed it especially for the wedding ceremony. Under this tent, the groom is surrounded by his family and best male friends. Female henna artists, called *tchinaden*, cover both his hands up to his wrists and his feet above his ankles with a solid non-decorative application of henna paste. His hands and feet are then wrapped in palm fronds and covered with plastic for a few hours. At this point the wrapping is removed and a beautiful bright orange hue is left to protect the groom from evil spirits for weeks.

YEMEN

During the Jewish wedding ceremony in Yemen, a ball of henna is placed in the tender hands of the bride and groom. Holding hands, they dance around the wedding circle. Then, as their hennaed hands touch in faithful union filled with love, they become husband and wife. The henna will stain their hands for a few weeks. After the wedding, with each glance at their hands, they are invited to remember this precious moment.

As people moved from place to place, traveling along the ancient trade routes, their stories, their customs and their seeds traveled with them. Families mingled over the centuries and marriages between tribes occurred. Customs blended and mixed and combined in new ways. Each family varied the style of the common traditions just as we personalize our celebrations.

MOROCCO

In Morocco, henna design has not only been used for weddings and beautification. It has also been a part of religious and cultural ceremonies for centuries. Here, the number seven has auspicious meaning. If a pregnant woman receives a henna design on her belly in her seventh month of pregnancy, this welcome distraction will also be a wish for good luck and a safe birth. It becomes a prayer for a healthy baby.

PAKISTAN

In Pakistan, it is believed that when the pregnant mother goes into labor it is good luck to have a henna design drawn upon her belly. This ensures that the mother will enter heaven as a bride, if by chance she does not make it through the labor. Henna is also used to color the hands and feet of infant boys at the time of circumcision. Births, birthdays and naming ceremonies are times henna designs abound.

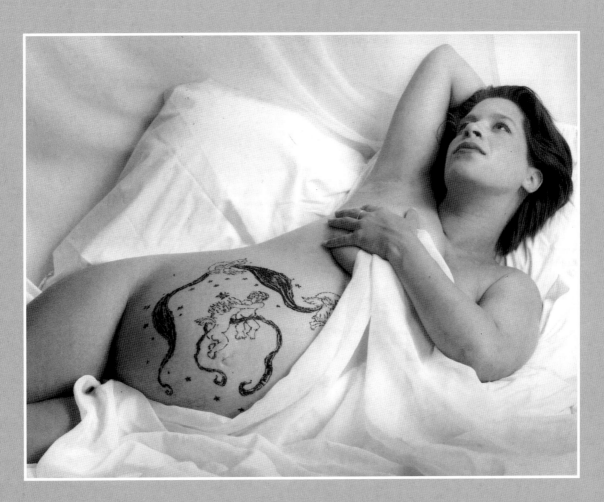

I am the womb where life begins and the breasts that nurture.

ISABEL ALLENDE

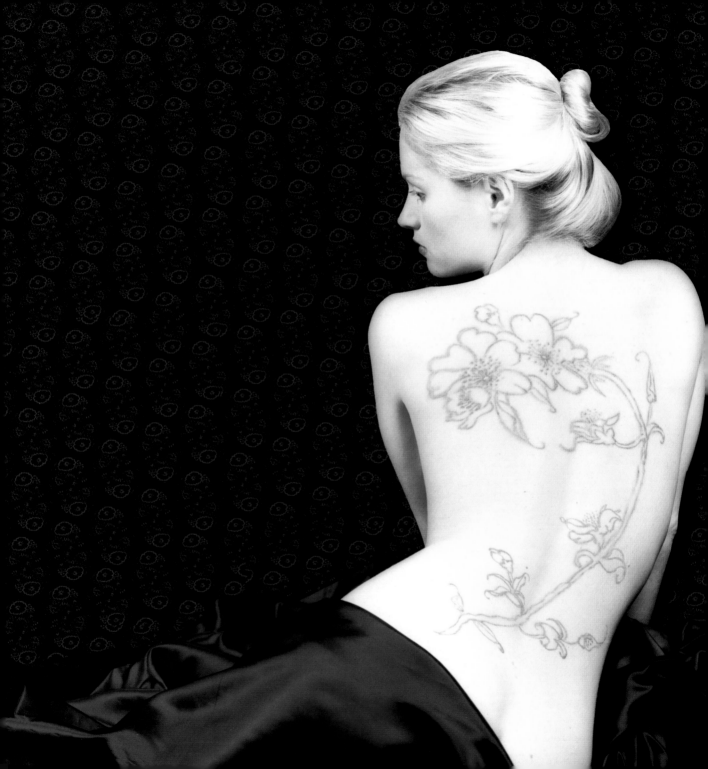

INDIA

Henna cannot be used during times of mourning in India because it is associated with celebration. At the Abrth-Indian festival of Kava-Chauth wives fast and henna their hands and feet in hopes the gods and goddesses will bestow their husbands long healthy lives. For certain festivals henna is used to dye the hooves and manes of horses. Elephants are decorated with beautiful orange henna to compliment hanging beaded tassels and brightly colored fabric.

EGYPT

In modern Egypt henna continues to be a very popular dye for fingernails and toenails. It is common to see the fingers stained up to the first joint and the palms of the hands or the soles of the feet intricately designed. It is still believed that the henna stain protects the skin from the elements. Egyptian women know, as did their ancestors, how to achieve a perfect black stain. They wait until the henna paste falls off then immediately apply a mixture of quicklime, ashes and linseed oil. It will blacken, as it has always done.

Henna has transcended political boundaries. Men and countries could go to war, but on both sides of the battle women were using henna. Henna has been used for centuries by people thousands of miles from one other. They use it for the same reasons of beautification and empowerment and for similar ceremonies. Henna has transcended all religions whether Hindu, Muslim, Sikh, Christian or Pagan. Women, men and children have all used henna—for love, for remembrance, for blessings, for pure joy and for the fun of it.

◄ *Flowers can be an evocative adornment.*

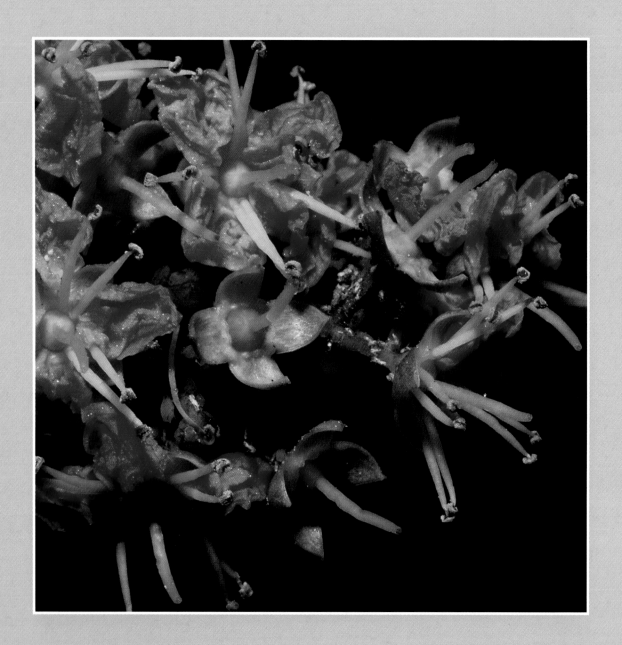

THE PLANT

In Egypt, henna is called Khenna, its Arabic name is Al Khanna, its Indian name is Mehendi. In England it is called Egyptian privet, in the West Indies where it is naturalized it is called Jamaica mignonette. It is called Henna in the United States and Europe, and the Berber people call it Ihenni. Other common names are Henne, Al-henna, Kihidab, Smooth lawsonis and Reseda. Henna is cultivated in the Middle East, India, Pakistan, Morocco, Iran, Australia, China, England and France.

The word henna evokes a world of beauty, leisure and sensuality. The henna plant however is a plain and common garden shrub grown in hot, usually dry but sometimes humid climates. It can grow from 6 to 25 feet, making it a good shade tree. Usually, however, it is cut to the size of a garden shrub. It bears large clusters of small fragrant white, yellow or rose colored flowers used for perfume and oils. Henna berries are used in medicinal mixtures.

This scrubby shrub, though cultivated in some regions, also can grow wild. In North Africa the seedlings are raised and will flourish about 12 years. The crop is cut down just above the ground twice a year to produce large quantities of leaf foliage for harvest. There are 55 to 60 species of henna, all of which have flowers that are used as dye.

Henna is traditionally valued for its use in creating beauty. It has strong dying qualities. A woman from Mauritius Island told me that when she was a little girl, she and her brothers and sisters would pick the

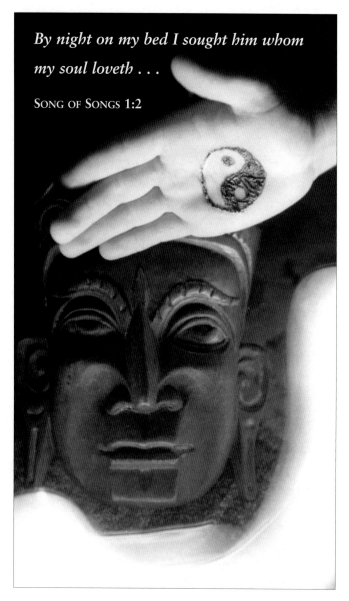

By night on my bed I sought him whom my soul loveth . . .

SONG OF SONGS 1:2

green leaves of the henna right off the tree. They would crush the leaves and add water. With this juice and using a small twig they would draw designs on each other just for fun. These designs would last several days.

There are so many different uses of henna—and often different plant varieties are used to suit the different purposes to which this versatile, magic plant is put. For example, the variety commonly used for staining the body and hair is:

> Botanical family:
> N.O. *Lythraceae*

> Botanical name:
> *Lawsonis inermis* and
> *Lawsonis alba*

The variety used for perfume is:

> Botanical family:
> *Resedaceae*

> Botanical name:
> *Reseda odorata*

Origins of Henna

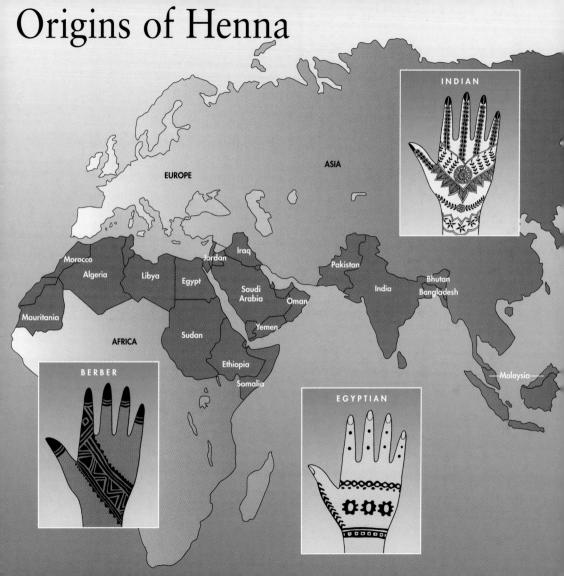

INDIAN

EUROPE

ASIA

Morocco
Algeria
Libya
Egypt
Jordan
Iraq
Pakistan
Bhutan
Bangladesh
India
Saudi
Arabia
Oman
Mauritania
AFRICA
Sudan
Yemen
Ethiopia
Somalia

BERBER

EGYPTIAN

Malaysia

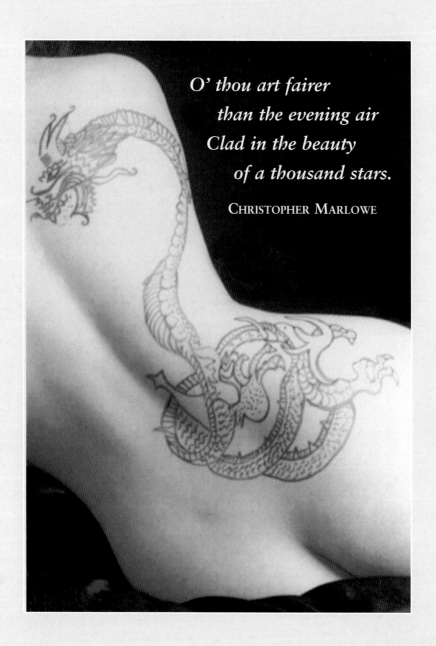

*O' thou art fairer
than the evening air
Clad in the beauty
of a thousand stars.*

CHRISTOPHER MARLOWE

The following quote from the *Art of Rajasthan* is an old advertisement for henna describing it as a magic cure-all for every kind of body and soul ailment. Substitute if you will the codliver oil your mother may have spooned you or vitamin C, the modern day remedy for complaints. This is how the old text reads:

Mehendi will give a new red color to one's unstable fortune and changes the course of fate. . . . It removes fatigue, cools the brain, and cures epilepsy when applied to the soles of the feet. When applied to hands, it sharpens the intellect and makes one think properly. Mehendi acts as an ointment on wounds, and when applied to the chest during the summer season, it keeps one cool and fresh for one week. One application cures boils. Tie a mehendi plaster around the joints of a horse's legs, and he will go four to five hundred miles without feeling fatigue. A bandage of mehendi cures the severest of headaches. Once dyed with mehendi, a white horse is infused with all the noble characteristics of a black horse. Anyone affected by an evil spirit is cured by the mehendi talisman, and if your wives' hands are decorated once a week, they'll need no guards nor chains to keep them in the harem. Mehendi turns gray hair black and infuses youth in old men.

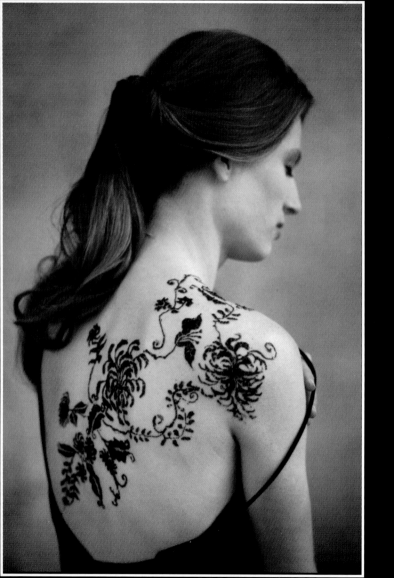

*I have gazed
at your beauty
from the beginning
of my existence . . .
Yet it has not been
long enough
for me.*

RABINDRANATH
TAGORE

AROMATHERAPY

In my experience, henna has an aromatherapy quality that elevates the mood, relaxing people instantly. In ancient Egypt, henna was used in the form of an essential oil. The medical book *Ebers Papyrus* described how henna is mixed with 16 oils to make a healing formula called *Kyphi*. This essential oil formula was burned in vessels over hot coals at sunset in honor of the sun god Ra. It is said to have a wonderful scent and also to be very tranquilizing. I can picture the woman lighting the incense to evoke a mood of quiet for her family, settling down with them after a meal of pears, almonds and gabgu-bird baked in a clay oven.

MEDICINAL USES

In the Middle East, henna is mixed with water and applied to the skin to kill lice, scabies and mange. It is also used to relieve itchy skin. For centuries people have rubbed henna on their scalps to keep their hair from falling out.

In Iran, a henna poultice is applied to relieve the pain of sprains and sore muscles.

In India, henna is mixed with ghee. This salve reduces the swelling of an injury.

In Yemen, when a child has a fever, a paste of henna is mixed into a ball and placed in the child's hand. This cools the young child's body bringing the temperature back down to normal.

◄ *Design inspried from an embroidered silk fabric from China.*

In Morocco, the women appreciate the soothing effect of henna on dry skin. They apply it to their hands and feet which are so often in water. Their skin becomes smooth and soft from this henna application. When henna flowers are mixed with vinegar and applied to the head it relieves headaches.

In some countries, the fruit of the henna tree is used to stimulate menstrual flow. Henna leaves help with fungal infections of the skin. People have stated that when using henna they have felt better, especially if they were tired, sick or nervous. Tamil physicians of southern India make an extract from the flowering twigs and leaves as an alternative therapy for leprosy.

Ayurvedic medicine has used henna to stimulate sexual desire.

When henna is applied to the head it is believed to enhance the sexual drive. This may well be the reason why people have a special henna ritual just before the wedding—to increase the pleasure on their wedding night.

HENNA FOR THE HAIR

Women and men throughout the modern and primitive worlds have used henna as a natural colorant for the hair. The stain from henna coats the outer layer of the hair follicle. The Romans and the Egyptians used henna to color their hair. Archaeologists have found mummies wrapped in henna-dyed cloth whose hair and beards were colored with henna.

In Morocco the ancient Berber people loved to color their hair with henna. They mixed henna powder with milk, eggs and the pulp of fruit to acquire a vibrant red.

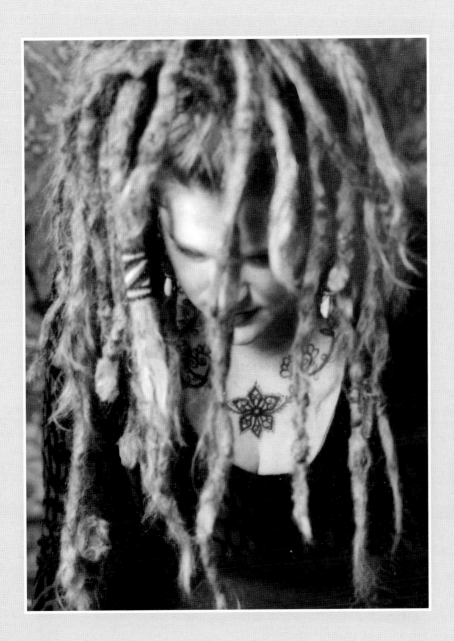

When I go
I will give
you surely

What you
will wear
if you go
with me;

A blanket
of red and
a bright girdle,

Two new
moccasins and
a silver necklace,

When I go
I will give
you surely

What you will
wear if you go
with me!

NORTH AMERICAN
INDIAN COURT-
SHIP SONG

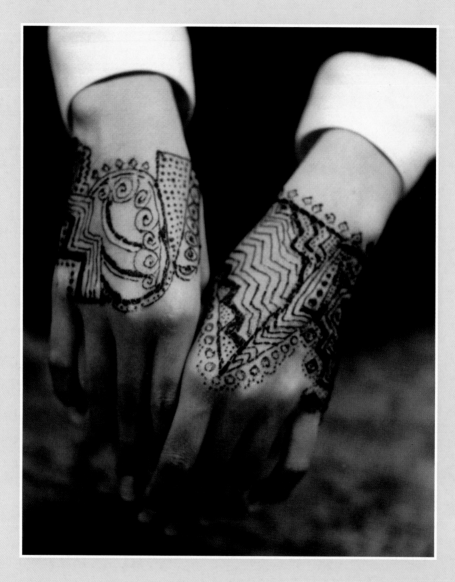

I am the hands that plow, and weave, and rock the child.

ISABEL ALLENDE

The henna that is used for the hair is the same henna that is used to decorate the skin. It is ground to a coarser powder and comes from the leaves that are harvested from the bottom of the henna plant. The leaves grown at the top of the plant are saved for use on the skin because they have the strongest staining ability. Hair henna has an inferior dying quality which makes it inadvisable to use for skin decoration. It also usually contains additives that might be harmful to the skin.

An unmarried man in India who has a little gray hair and wants to get married is encouraged, usually by his mother, to henna his hair. This is done by applying a paste in the hair for several hours a week. After a month or two the stain becomes such a dark red that it will blend very well with the rest of his hair. Then he may be more marriageable.

In ancient Morocco, the prophet Mohammed used henna to stain his beard a lovely red color. He believed the henna plant had mystical and magical powers. The people of Morocco listened to him and began calling henna "The Light of the Prophet" from that time, and the henna plant became embedded in tradition. Even today men in Morocco follow this powerful tradition and color their beards and hair with henna.

Henna arrived in America in the 1930's during the Great Depression as hair coloring. Natural ingredients such as powdered indigo leaves, ground cloves or coffee were added to the henna to darken it. Today henna has blended with technology. Various metallic salts are added to produce colors other than red.

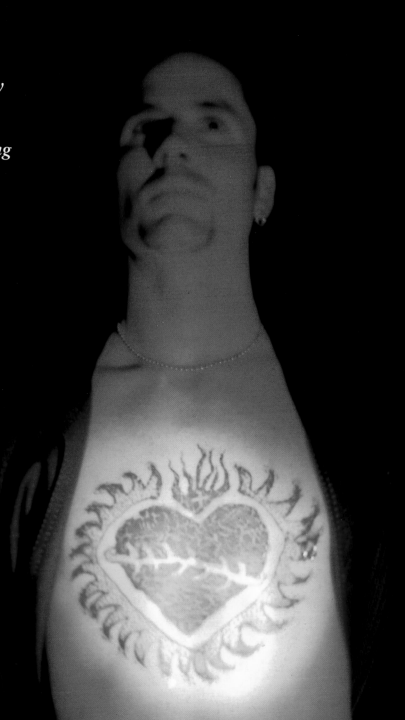

*The true
revolutionary
is guided by
a great feeling
of love.*

CHE GUEVARA

PERFUME

For centuries henna flowers have been used for perfume. Several species have very fragrant blossoms. They emit a wonderful scent reminiscent of the lilac. During the time of the Middle Kingdom in Egypt, and again in Rome, henna perfumed graves and tombs. In beautiful bottles and jars of alabaster, glass, ivory, onyx, or bone, safely and secretly stored for centuries, exquisite remnants of these oils scented with the blooms of henna have been found. I imagine a lady of long ago, waiting for her lover. She places scented oil on her wrists, filling the balmy night air with this sweet aroma. Wonderfully scented oils served as potions to cleanse the body—a welcome expression in the hot dry climate of Egypt where soap was yet to be invented.

MEN AND HENNA

Henna has traveled over centuries and over continents. It has adorned the hands and arms of voluptuous women and the callused feet of the Tuareg men from the Sahara desert. Now that henna has arrived on the shores of the North American continent, the great blending pot, it is being transformed once again. Many men find themselves intrigued with the juices of the henna plant—they are becoming henna artists.

I've asked all the men I've hennaed what it meant for a man to want a henna design. I felt their reactions perhaps stemmed from ancient roots and tribal beginnings, when "coming of age" for a young boy was always celebrated. In those days, males were tattooed in groups. Gathering together gave them strength and valor which galvanized their spirits. Later they would mark their bodies for good luck and, together, go into battle. These were rites of initiation.

We have so few rites or rituals in our culture to meet this need of marking a moment of passage or completion or belonging. A hennaed symbol on the body can connect us to our past.

Today boys can get a henna design when a permanent tattoo is not available. Or a man can try out a design prior to getting a permanent tattoo. Getting a henna design can renew his virile nature, his creativity, his individuality and at the same time satisfy a drive to be a part of something. It is an opportunity for him to express himself. He can be a rebel without alienation.

Henna provides a nonverbal way to make a statement. Nothing much has changed over the centuries except the symbols—and most of those have remained the same. Men still have a basic drive to mark their bodies. This ancient body art serves that urge whether it be to denote bravery, strength, courage, virility or a tribal connection. And why not? Most people, particularly women, will find a hennaed man erotic, sexy, bold and physical. These are the men of the new tribe.

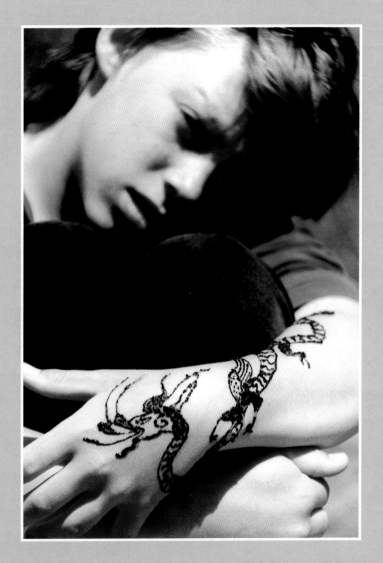

Life is the most wonderful fairy tale.

HANS CHRISTIAN ANDERSON

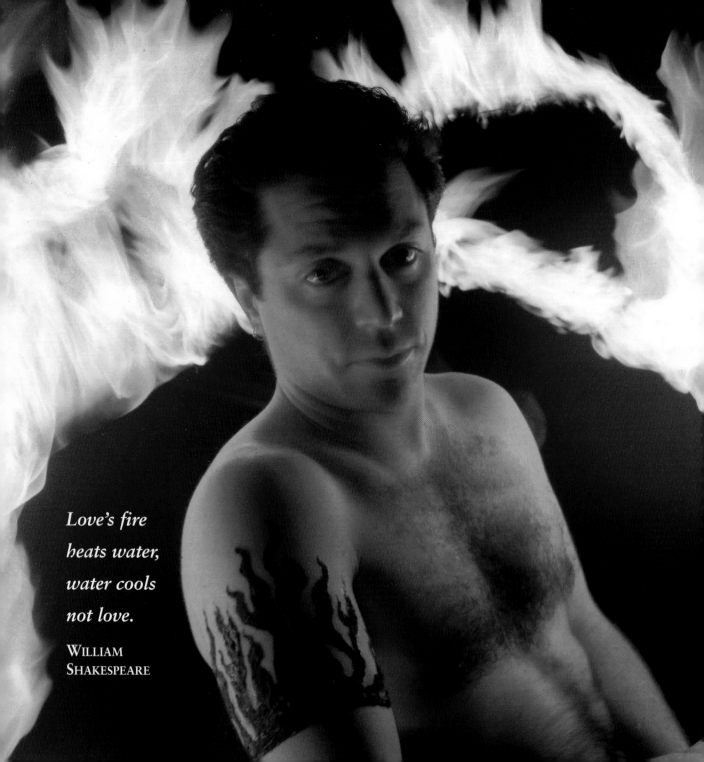

*Love's fire
heats water,
water cools
not love.*

WILLIAM
SHAKESPEARE

J have been bewitched and seduced by henna, the ultimate aphrodisiac and supreme nurturing mother plant. Henna nurtures my body as a gateway to my dreams and has served this divine function through all time. Henna heals wandering souls in exotic secret salons in Morocco. Henna brings sick bodies back to life in North American hospitals when applied as a symbol and talisman of hope and love.

As we turn to forms of healing other than the antiseptic, sterile hospital bed and technological solutions offered by modern medicine, people more and more look to the heavens for healing and to ancient plant remedies, whose healing properties are being rediscovered today. Henna merges both.

For centuries the henna plant has taken the role of healer, weaving together spirit, body and culture. From roots in ancient traditions the spirit of henna has been passed to modern life. Partakers have used henna for many different kinds of occasions but the outcome is always profound.

Henna can be very healing for the person who is physically ill. I place a meaningful mandala design on a person as a good luck charm to fill them with hope and protection. One of my dearest friends was near death. I hennaed a heart on his hand to remind him of my love for him. It lasted all the while he convalesced. Another time a very special woman had one of her breasts removed due to cancer. She asked me to henna a phoenix bird onto her scar. This very powerful symbol of rebirth and healing helped her transform her experience in a very positive way.

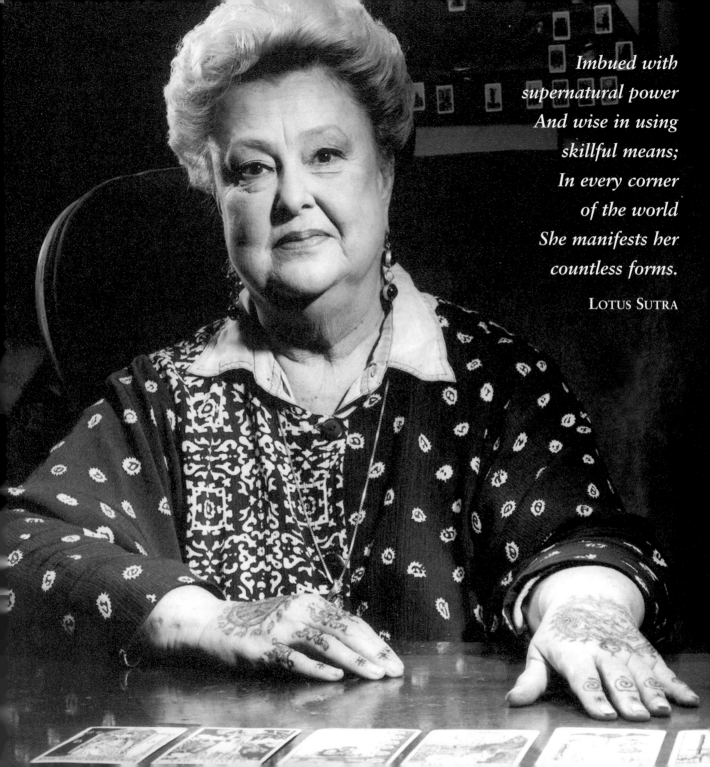

*Imbued with
supernatural power
And wise in using
skillful means;
In every corner
of the world
She manifests her
countless forms.*

LOTUS SUTRA

Our vibration changes when we wear henna designs. Henna brings such joy and laughter into all our lives. This raises our endorphin levels. Generous endorphin levels stimulate the healing process. This is a well-known medical fact.

Healing is also spiritual and communal. I have used it at many kinds of healing workshops as a tool for transformation. Henna is valuable to use in preparation for a time of change such as graduation from school, a birth, a death or a divorce. In our culture we need external support for life's many ups and downs. We need to mark the significant moments of passage to help us through and to celebrate. Henna has always been a generous and beautiful goddess of healing. For centuries now she makes herself available to us. She blends into our very pores. She lends us her power of beauty and hope. And we laugh, and we heal.

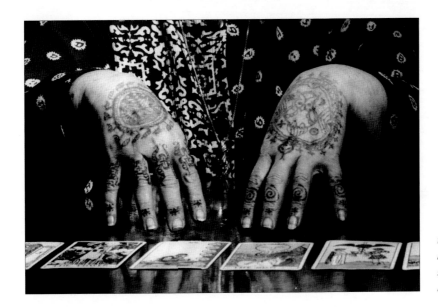

◄ *There are many symbols in this design—the owl, the snake, a healing shield, a sacred spiral—representing strength and wisdom.*

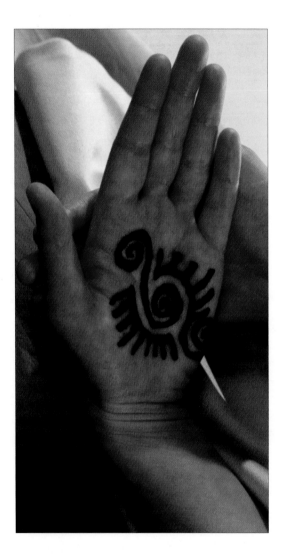

Mayan design with henna paste.

feet than on some other places of the body. The higher up you go on your arms and legs, the lighter the stain will be. For most people henna applied on the tummy, back and shoulders will also be a little lighter.

In all the world, you are unique. Despite all the rules we use to apply henna, the surprise will come as your body interacts with the henna.

WHAT COLOR WILL MY DESIGN BE?

Your skin will stain from a deep orange to dark reddish brown. Once again, it depends on the tone of the skin. Most of the time people with lighter skin will stain in the brown tones while people with darker skin will stain in more of the deep orange tones. If you are a dark skinned person, you may need to apply the henna twice to obtain a deep stain. But there are always exceptions. That's the wonder of it.

Some say the darker the design, the stronger your love. And, of course, if it doesn't turn out, just reapply.

If you buy henna and your skin turns a color other than reddish brown or deep orange, it means there are additives in the product.

Henna artists throughout the world have found many interesting ways to get a dark stain. For instance, in Morocco holding the hands and feet over a flattened pan containing smoking cloves has been known to turn the design black. In the Sudan the henna artists will hold the henna design over a fire. When the design has been smoked just enough the henna paste is brushed off and from the embers arises a brilliant midnight black motif. This is called *dukhan*. Adding rose petal tea to the henna has been known to captivate the paste in such a way that it adds a slight red color to the stain. It also makes for a wonderful scent.

I've also heard over the henna grapevine that black walnut, hemp and fresh-crushed leaves of indigo give a black to bluish-black dye. You may want to experiment. Try it and let me know.

How Long Will a Henna Design Last?

The stain will last the longest in the spots it dyes the darkest. For example, a henna stain can last from 2 to 4 weeks on the hands and feet, and 1 to 2 weeks on other places. The design will start to fade as the epidermal cells replenish themselves. Going to the spa, visiting the hot tub or steam room frequently, swimming, gardening and having your hands in water regularly will wear off your henna design quickly.

You can protect the design somewhat by moistening your skin with olive or almond oil. Can you imagine how good this feels?

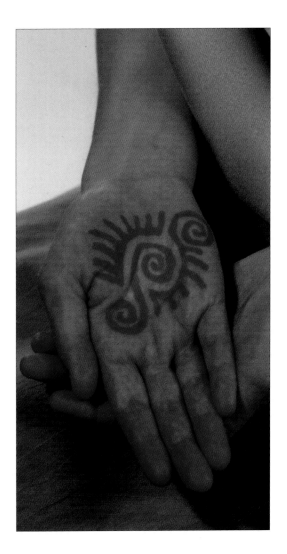

Mayan design one day after the removal of paste.

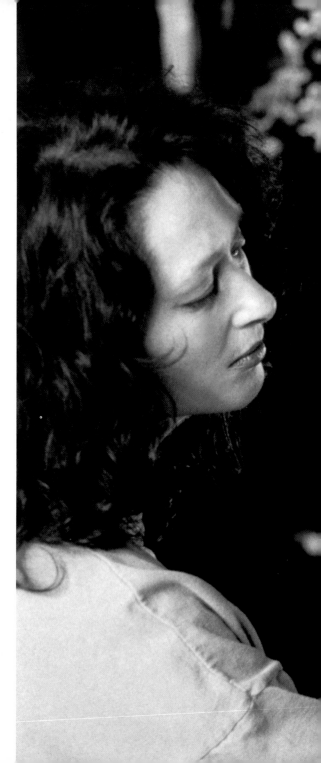

The henna ritual is especially wonderful for both the one receiving the design and the artist applying it. As the henna artist, you will want to create a comfortable environment for both of you. Remember that henna designing can take from 20 minutes to more than 5 hours to complete, depending on the complexity of the design. I always gather up as many pillows, cushions and pads as possible. I put them everywhere—behind backs, under feet, under elbows. Help the person receiving the design settle into a good position. Find the right chairs or places to sit. Sometimes it is best to sit on the floor. For yourself, be sure your back is supported and there is a place to rest your arm or elbow. You won't want to lean over or strain yourself.

For the one receiving the design, it is really important that you wear clothing which is going to free up the body for the design. Tight jeans can be difficult to get off if the feet or ankles are freshly hennaed. Putting on a jacket over the hands or arms can be tricky. So plan ahead. Generally speaking, loose clothing is the best.

To help evoke a peaceful atmosphere, you may wish to have on hand some incense and your favorite music. Warm tea and simple food are also wise preparations.

▸ *Applying henna with a bottle.*

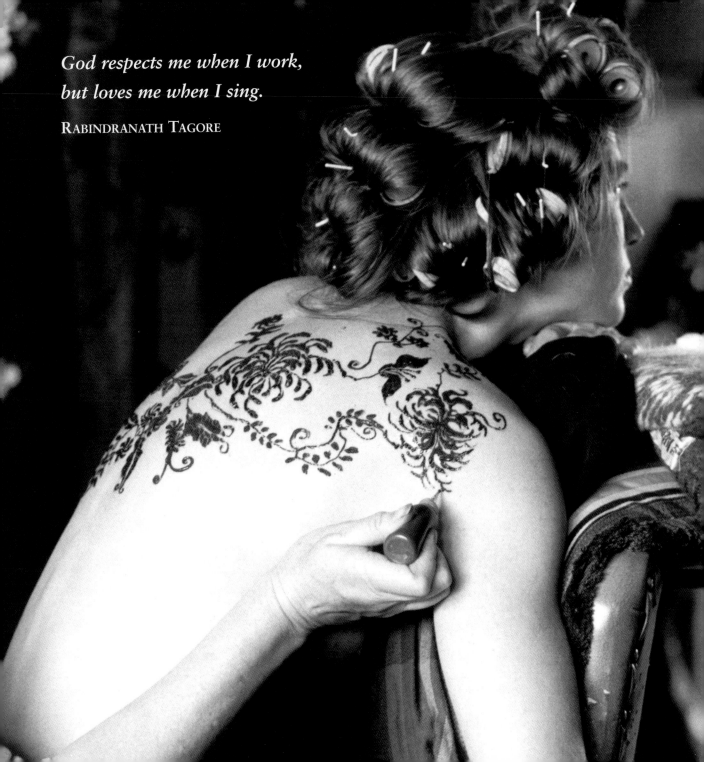

God respects me when I work,
but loves me when I sing.

RABINDRANATH TAGORE

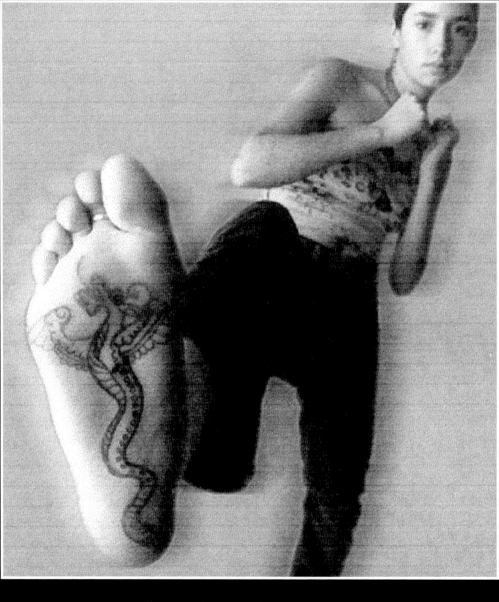

Love rules without rules. ITALIAN PROVERB

Follow your instincts. Think about your design and which part of your body you want adorned. You get to choose. Hands and feet are very good places, because this is where you will get your darkest stain. The henna paste must remain on the skin for 6 to 12 hours, so putting designs in places that might rub against the body, like the inside of the arm or on your back, will take extra planning. Watch out for shoe straps and watchbands that may touch the henna design. They can wear it off very quickly.

The bottoms of the feet are a beautiful place for a henna design, but find a nice comfortable reclining chair because you will not be able to walk while the henna is curing. Take care of those bathroom visits in advance.

I always prefer to receive my henna designs in the evening so I can sleep with the paste on and not have to worry about disturbing the design. Some people wrap their feet and hands in cotton fabric to further protect the design and anything it may touch.

Placing the henna on the neck, shoulders and chest elicits a particular kind of beautiful design, especially if the right piece of clothing is worn to show it off like a piece of jewelry. For instance, an attractive necklace or a symbol can be very appealing. Just think, a chance to wear jewelry you need not remove. However, since the skin is thinner in these places the design will not be as dark and will last only between 1 to 1 1/2 weeks.

Putting a design on the stomach area is great especially during the summer months when it can be seen. On the stomach, henna can last between 1 to 2 weeks.

Placing henna in the hidden places can be an arousing and pleasant surprise. For instance lovely designs on the breasts, upper thighs and genital area are sometimes done for the wedding night or a rendezvous with your sweetheart. In these areas the henna will last between 1 to 2 weeks.

And, of course, consider a design on the hands. No menial chores should be done while henna is on your hands. In India women are not to do housework as long as you can see lines of the henna design. Good reason to apply and reapply! Applying a henna design might be temporarily inconvenient, but be patient. Be adventurous. The results will be worth it. The main thing is to enjoy, listen to music, feast and maybe just do nothing for awhile. It is good for your soul.

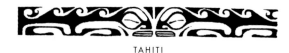

TAHITI

FIJI

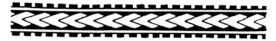

SAMOA

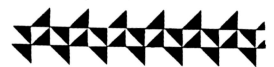

TONGA

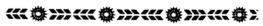

HAWAII

NEW HEBRIDES

BANDS

There are so many choices when it comes to picking the right henna design. In fact, it can seem impossible to decide. Take a chance and pick a design you really like. Henna designs are temporary, so you can plan on having many more.

To help you in your search I have included a group of designs I've collected from many cultures *(pp. 80–123)*. Some are simple to draw and some are more complicated. If you are just beginning, you can start with the simple ones. As you gain more confidence, try the ones that are more complicated.

Henna designs throughout time have reflected peoples' lifestyles. They would express themselves through henna designs drawn from reflections, impressions and experiences in their daily lives. For instance, an intricately designed Persian rug or tapestry from one of the Middle Eastern countries certainly inspired many a henna artist. Or did the henna artist inspire the weaver? Embroideries, lace, jewelry and nature are all perfect places to get ideas for henna designs. If you find a design you like, but it seems too difficult or too large, it is possible to modify the design by just using a small part of it as your final pattern. Be adventurous! Surrender yourself to this lovely practice discovered by Venus herself.

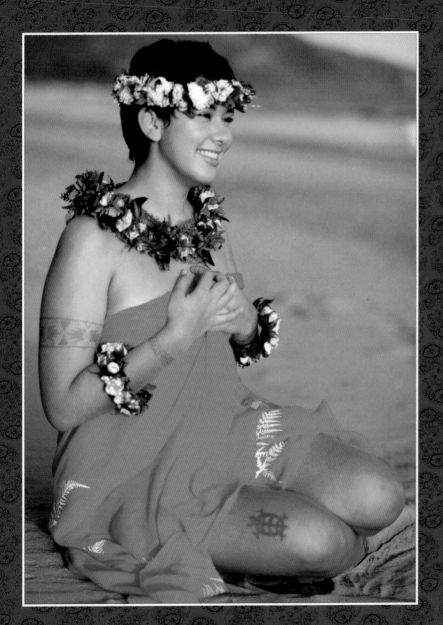

Listen to me sweet breeze

Companion of mine

And what do you think

you're doing

Dodging away from me

Oh you Pu'ulena wind.

HAWAIIAN SONG
MOANIKE'ALA
PRINCE LELEIOHOKU

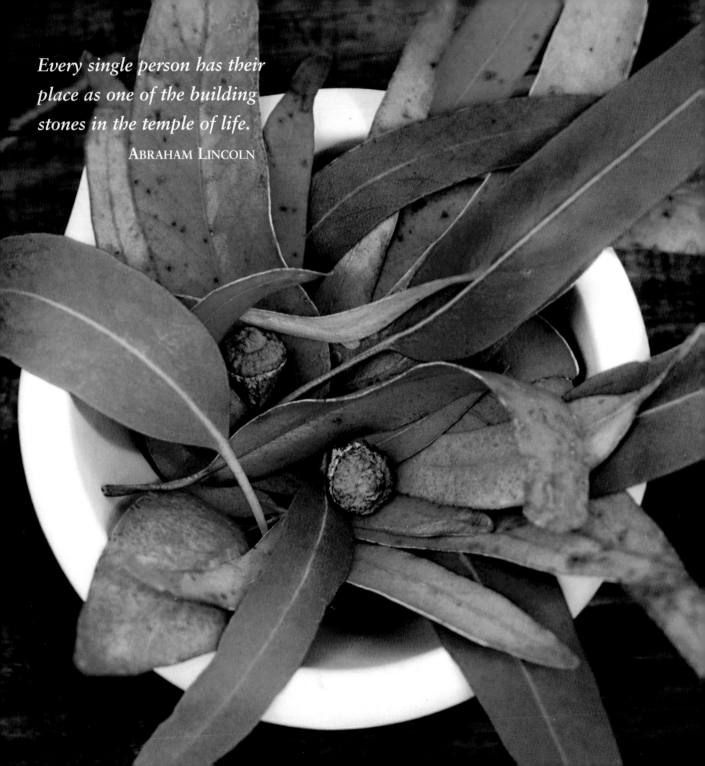

Every single person has their place as one of the building stones in the temple of life.

ABRAHAM LINCOLN

Cleansing and preparing the skin is a vital part of the henna process. Traditionally in many other cultures, this step of bathing and purification has sometimes taken several days. Adequate skin preparation will insure a longer life to the design and almost always a darker color. Cleopatra liked to clean and soften her skin with a mixture of honey and ground almonds. Julius Caesar and Marc Antony could not resist her. I know my experience with men has revealed that henna has an erotic effect on them that defies the conscious mind. There is something tantalizing and arousing about a woman adorned with henna on her glowing skin. Cleopatra knew this. So think royally. Your skin is your ultimate earth treasure.

Skin preparation must be done the day before or it will interfere with the staining process. So plan a good block of uninterrupted time in the henna

◄ *Oil from eucalyptus leaves is often used in henna paste.*

tradition. Find a nice exfoliating cream, gel or loofah sponge and gently remove dead cells from the surface of the skin. If you have chosen a place that has some hair growth, you can shave off the hair 24 hours before getting the design, although this isn't always necessary. Make sure all soap and shaving cream is removed hours before application. You might make a potion of natural scents placed in water. Use this aromatic balm to gently cleanse the area chosen for designs.

Some say if you apply a light coat of pre-opening oil such as clove, olive, almond or mehlabiya oil, it helps to make the design darker. Mehlabiya oil is a mixture of oils and herbs that can be purchased at an Indian store that specializes in imports. Massaging in a light coat of pre-opening oil may be helpful in some skin types. Be careful, some mixtures might have chemical additives.

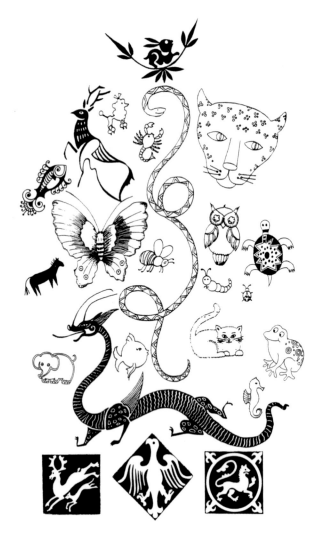

When you have finished applying the design you must leave the henna paste on the skin for 6 to 12 hours. The longer you can leave the design on, the longer it will last. This is your time to plan to relax. You will emerge transformed.

The next step is as magical as it is mysterious. One minute you will go to sleep with the design a light faint color. By the second morning when you wake up it will have changed into a rich mahogany hue, much darker and more pronounced. Don't get discouraged when you wake that first morning if it appears not to be staining. The henna is still at work.

How does this happen? It is called "curing." Even if I do this a thousand times I still am amazed at the mystery of henna. After the henna is applied to the skin, it takes 2 to 3 days to reach its darkest color. If the design is on the light side, don't worry. Just reapply the henna for more dramatic results.

If you are in bright sunshine while you have a henna design, you can get a reverse tan. The skin under the henna stain will remain lighter because the henna stain acts as a sun block. You may want to play with this idea.

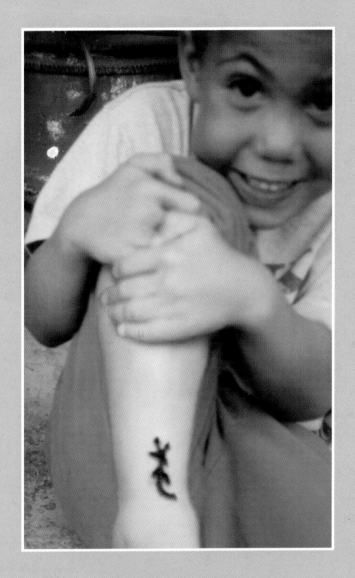

Be aware of your dreams, they just might come true.

JEWISH PROVERB

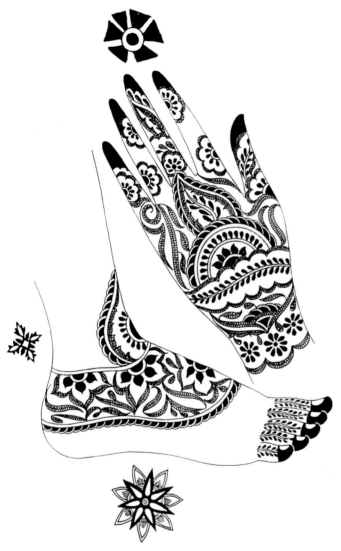

INDIA

SIFTING THE POWDER

The next step is to sift the henna powder. This part of the henna process must be done well. So here is another chance to relax, daydream and just melt away to other worlds. Place a piece of loosely woven fabric across the mouth of a jar or bowl. Hold the fabric with one hand and move a spoon back and forth over the henna on the fabric. The sifted powder will fall through the cloth and leave small pieces of the stems and larger henna particles. Throw these away. Do this two or three times. If you don't want to sift henna, you can purchase pre-sifted henna from companies that import henna products.

Sifting the henna and making a smooth paste are a very important part of henna designing. This I cannot emphasize enough. Carefully mixed paste will please the "henna gods" and enable you to draw intricate patterns with fine lines of henna, without clogging the plastic cone or bottle.

PRE-MIXED HENNA IN TUBES

Clearly it is best to mix your own henna paste. However, using a tube can be very convenient and a good initial step in learning the art of henna. There are many tubes on the market but only a few are of high quality. The staining ability of the pre-mixed henna in tubes can vary depending on the strength of that particular henna. Tubes can provide enough paste for 10 to 12 small designs and 2 to 4 large intricate designs. There is a mild preservative added to the paste, so a securely capped tube can last several months. If this is not done, the henna will become dry and lose its dying quality. It is always best to test the henna paste on the skin before you do a design, although allergic reactions to henna or the preservatives are rare. Do not get henna near the eyes or open wounds. You can have a professional design in minutes if the henna is pre-mixed. I have included a pre-mixed tube in this kit to encourage everyone, including children, to give it a try.

My friend in New York, an innovative teacher of eight-year-olds, recently handed a tube to each one of his 20 students. To his surprise they knew exactly what to do. They covered each other's hands with delightful designs and a good time was had by all.

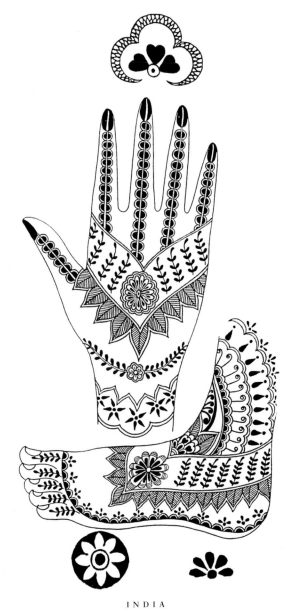

INDIA

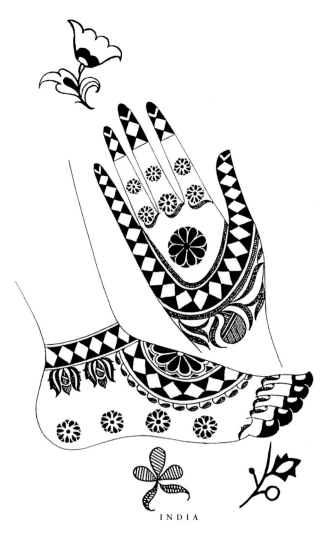

INDIA

1. Choose the right size plastic tip and place it on the tube. Tips are included in the box.

2. Squeeze out the henna paste from the tube onto the skin in the form of a design. There are many wonderful designs from which to choose right in this book.

3. For even faster results, squeeze the henna onto a stencil to get a professional looking design in minutes.

THE HENNA PASTE

Throughout the world, henna artists have captured the spirit and power of henna by making henna paste in many different ways. Artists have experimented, applied and re-applied until they came up with marvelous results.

Henna is very easy to mix because most of the ingredients are already in your kitchen. The most common ingredients used are black tea, coffee, lemons, limes, cloves, sugar, eucalyptus oil, glycerine and water. Some of the more exotic ingredients that can be used are tamarind, cardamom, methys seeds (fenugreek), betel leaves, turmeric, saffron, rose petals and orange blossom water. In India, young girls on street corners near bustling marketplaces make wonderfully majestic henna designs for a small price. Their henna paste is mixed only in water. The designs last for weeks. Their sweetness lasts forever.

Water is a very simple but very important ingredient. I always use spring or rain water in mixing henna paste. When I first began drawing henna designs I noticed they were not lasting long enough. I discovered it was because I was using water from my tap which is unfiltered and chemically treated. By simply switching to spring water, my designs became strong and vibrant.

Mixing the henna paste takes a little practice but it is easy to do. I like to use a plastic bowl to mix the paste, although some prefer ceramic bowls. You will need to place the henna powder in your bowl and prepare to make the henna tea.

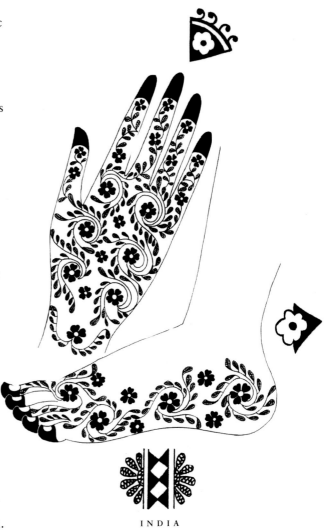

INDIA

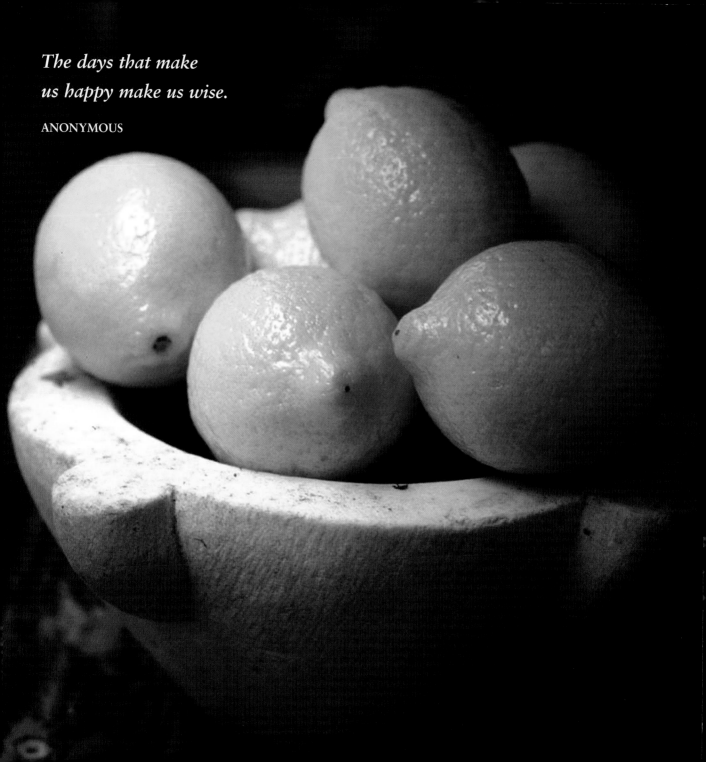

The days that make
us happy make us wise.

ANONYMOUS

The Henna Tea

The henna tea is the liquid that is added to the henna powder. The most common ingredients used in the henna tea are black tea, powdered cloves and tamarind. Cardamom, turmeric, coffee and saffron can also be used. These ingredients serve as colorants. Boil the ingredients until the tea is thick and has the consistency of syrup.

Now let it stand overnight. Invite the henna jinni to do their work. In the morning when you arise, heat up the henna tea again until it is warm. Strain it. While it is still very warm, mix and stir it with the powder. The heat sometimes helps to break down the powdered leaf to produce a better dye. After mixing it thoroughly you are now ready to add the mordant.

Your kitchen will be transformed with aromas of this fragrant henna-herbed tea. Don't forget—henna has an aromatherapy quality that will elevate your mood.

The Mordant

The mordant is an ingredient used to fix or activate the dying agent of henna. In other words, the mordant is the catalyst to bring out the passion of the color within the henna plant.

Lemon and lime juice are very good to use as mordants. Limes are my favorite. You can squeeze the juice of fresh limes, which is the best, or you can buy lime juice pre-squeezed at the grocery store. A strong mordant can be made by cutting a lime in slices and letting them dry. Then boil the dried lime slices until the water turns red. Use this lime water for the mordant.

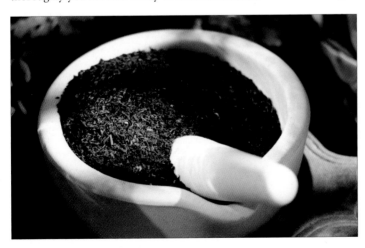

opposite: Lemons used in henna paste.
◄ *Black tea, an ingredient for henna paste.*

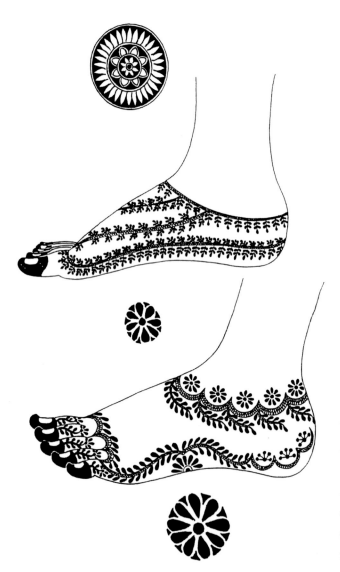

INDIA

If, in your henna travels, you find that your henna recipe is not quite doing what it is supposed to do, that the stains are not dark enough or they don't last long, just add lemon or lime juice and extra eucalyptus oil. Your problem might be solved. If the henna powder has been exposed to light or moisture, or if it is too old, this may not work. You will never know until you try. I have found that I am constantly surprised with henna. I love to play with these ingredients because I'm always trying to find the best henna recipes.

THE OIL

Next, you add the oil. I have a lot of success with eucalyptus oil. Clove, mustard and mehlabiya oil are also used. Be careful, however, as they can sometimes irritate the skin.

The oil plays an important role in the henna paste. It acts as an emollient binding the paste together so it will have a creamy smooth consistency. Other ingredients that have been used as emollients are eggs, sugar, sticky rice, and okra. If your paste is stiff and doesn't stick to the skin easily, it might need more oil. Mix in extra oil with a spoon. Blend and crush any lumps to get a good consistency.

MIXING THE PASTE

Good henna paste requires using the correct ingredients in their right proportions. Knowing when the paste is thoroughly mixed takes a little practice. But practice makes perfect. It can't be too runny or too dry. It should be creamy and similar to the consistency of icing for a cake. If you have ever mixed a batch of brownies or a cake from a mix, then you can make henna paste.

A good way to test the henna paste is to put a little line on your hand. Shake your hand. If the henna is runny, then the paste is too thin and needs more henna powder. If the paste doesn't adhere to the skin easily and is clumpy, the henna is too dry and needs more oil or tea.

Mix until you have a creamy consistency and all of the lumps are dissolved. Then add the lemon or lime juice and finally the eucalyptus oil. This takes a little practice but soon you will have your own compelling henna paste.

Stirring the paste mixture thoroughly and letting it stand for 12 to 48 hours yields the best results. If you have good henna powder, it will reach the height of its potency at 48 hours.

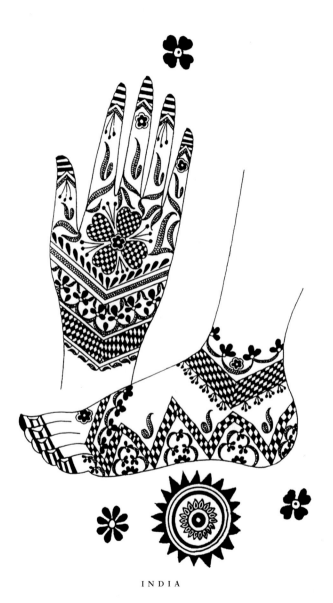

INDIA

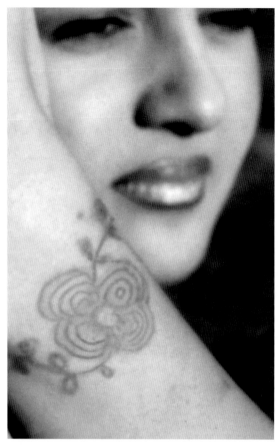

This was a design taken from her grandmother's Persian rug.

Sometimes, as a final step, I will strain the henna mixture through a fine tea strainer to catch any remaining henna particles, which I discard. This step ensures that the paste will not clog the cone or bottle, and will be easy to apply on the skin. I like to mix henna in the evening. By the morning it develops a glistening sheen. Then you know your henna particles have been transformed.

Keep the henna paste at room temperature so you don't disturb the development of the dye process. If you have sensitive skin, put a little on as a test to see if you have any adverse reactions. Also, always keep the paste away from the eyes or wounds.

Storing the Paste

Since henna paste must be made in advance, it is possible to store the henna by freezing it in a covered ice cube tray or in plastic for future use. Frozen henna will last up to two months. Refrigerated paste will last 3 to 4 days. Freeze or refrigerate only after the paste has reached full potency.

In the next section I have included a number of recipes, each different in their ingredients and in their cultural backgrounds. Give them a try. Find your favorites. Experiment and adjust the measurements. Make up your own elixirs. And don't forget, henna designing is an art, and there are many paths to beautiful henna designs.

Henna recipes are centuries old. They have been passed from one generation to another. Each recipe is soaked with its own magical essence and history arriving from henna kitchens everywhere. So gather up a bowl and a spoon. Be creative. Have fun. Try these different recipes and experience the results. You might find yourself falling in love with henna.

PAKISTANI RECIPE

2 tbsp. sifted henna powder
1 black tea bag
2 tsp. powdered cloves
1 tsp. white sugar
1 lemon or lime
10 drops eucalyptus oil
spring water

First make a tea by boiling the powdered cloves, black tea and the sugar and let cool. Then add very slowly, while stirring with a spoon, approximately one tablespoon of tea, one tablespoon of lemon or lime juice and ten drops of eucalyptus oil to two tablespoons of sifted henna. You can add extra henna or tea if needed. Mix until the mixture turns into a consistency similar to cake icing.

CHINA

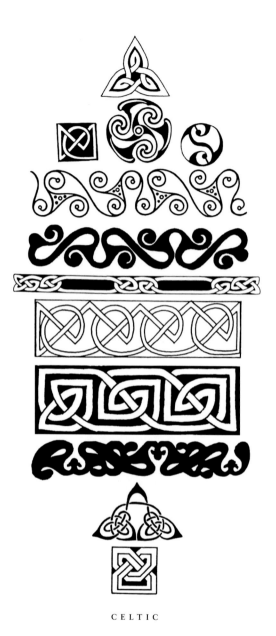

CELTIC

A Truly Simple Henna Recipe

This recipe is simple and reliable, especially if you are in a pinch for time. Gradually add lime or lemon juice and eucalyptus oil (double what you would normally use) to the henna powder. No need to add any other liquids. Mix until you get a creamy consistency. If your henna powder is good quality, you can get excellent results. Let it stand for 12 to 48 hours and put into a cone or bottle. If this fails, then the henna powder might be too old or it has lost its dying potential due to exposure to light, moisture or air.

East Indian Recipe from Henna FAQ

Boil 1/2 cup of purified water with 1 teaspoon of methys seeds (fenugreek) and 1 teaspoon black tea leaves. Leave uncovered. Let boil approximately 3-4 minutes until the water looks dark brown. Strain the water through a sieve. Let cool. Set seeds aside. If you dry these, you can reuse them a second time for boiling.

In a bowl, pour 1/2 cup water with 1 teaspoon sugar and 1/2 teaspoon tamarind paste. Let dissolve approximately 10 minutes. Do not boil. After a few minutes, combine both solutions and stir. There will be pieces floating around. Strain them as best you can through a fine sieve. Add 3 to 4 drops of eucalyptus oil to the solution. You can wear surgical gloves to avoid staining hands while working with the paste.

In a glass or plastic bowl, drop in 2 soft heaping teaspoons of sifted powder. Add 1 teaspoon of the tea/tamarind solution, stirring into the powder. You will need to add the water solution slowly to the powder to avoid making it too soupy. The paste will be the correct consistency when it looks like brownie batter—slightly stiff, doesn't run off the spoon, but has a moist sheen on it when left to sit for 5 to 10 seconds.

RAJASTHANI (NORTHERN INDIAN) RECIPE

1 black tea bag
2 tsp. tamarind paste
2 tsp. of coffee
2-3 tbsp. sifted henna powder
eucalyptus oil
clove oil

Simmer fitrst three ingredients in 2 cups of water for one hour. Let cool. Then add to henna powder slowly until mixture is like pancake batter. Let stand for several hours, then add 5 drops of eucalyptus oil and clove oil. Put into cones.

NORTH AFRICAN (MOROCCAN) RECIPE BY ME'IRA, KIM

1. Purchase fresh red powder henna (Afshan or Sadqu brands boxed and wrapped)

2. One cup brewed black tea, allowed to sit overnight

3. 1 teaspoon fresh lemon juice or a lemon which has sat in the sun for 12 hours or more.

4. Use a brass (not ceramic) bowl

5. Mixing spoon

6. Rose and orange water to wash hands and feet before application.

For application, the traditional North African tool is a Mishwak pick.

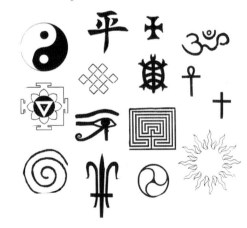

SYMBOLS

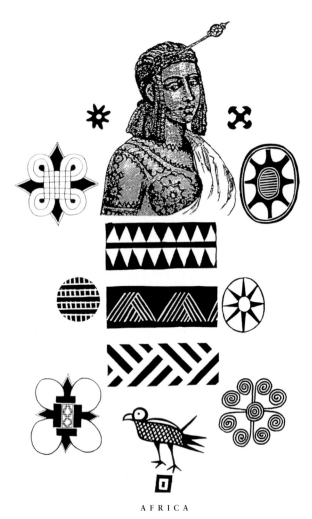

AFRICA

There are many ways to apply henna. Thousands of years ago people had time to feed their spirits by creating radiant art on each other's bodies. They would sit by the side of a fire or perhaps under the shade of a date palm tree and apply henna with little "toothpick"-like sticks. They could get very intricate results, but it did take time.

In Africa, a flattened stick with a little curve to it (similar to a spoon) was used to contain the henna as it was dripped in long lines across the tops and bottoms of the hands and feet to create geometric designs. With slivers of wood, the designs could be touched-up. Over time artists have come up with the most interesting ways to create irresistible henna designs.

My friends in New Delhi, India, told me that long ago henna artists would mix the henna paste into a very stringy, stretchy consistency similar to egg whites using extra amounts of the emollient herbs that I have mentioned in the section on oil. They would put this paste between their fingers then pull their fingers apart, and there would be a thin line of henna. They would then carefully lay this line on the most strategic place and begin to form the design.

Another method is to drip wax onto the skin in free flowing designs. When the wax has hardened, delicately spread the henna on top of the hardened wax. When it is time, flake off the henna. Remove the wax and marvelously the design will show up in skin tones. Because of the wax, the henna will stain all of the areas around the design leaving it free of henna. You get a design in reverse. If you do not want to use wax, a paste of lime can be used in its place.

I have also made reverse designs by covering an area with henna then scraping off the henna in strategic places to create a motif. If this is done at different times, you can get a finished design with varying intensities of color. Your result will be delightfully three dimensional.

Today henna artists have on hand Q-tips, cotton balls, flat toothpicks, tissue paper and a little water if necessary to touch up. Remember even the best henna artists make a mistake from time to time.

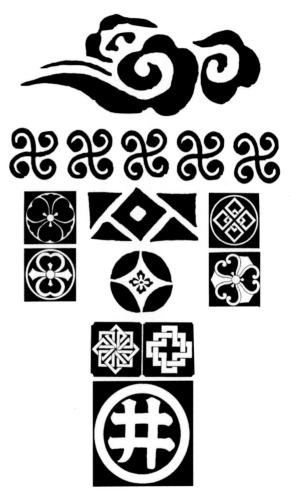

JAPAN

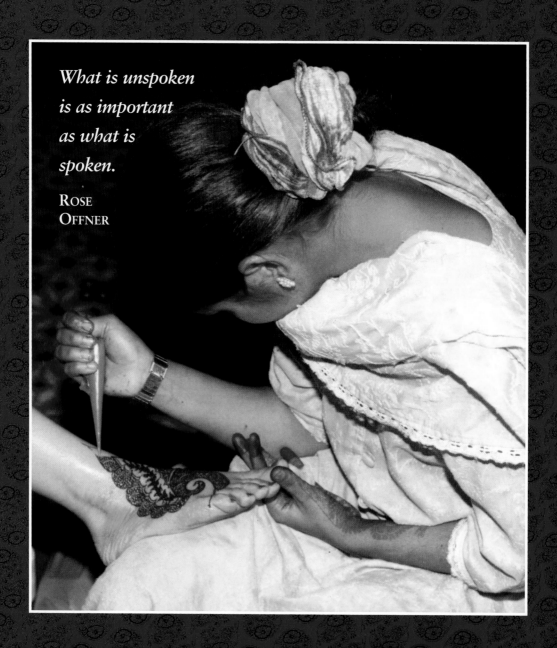

*What is unspoken
is as important
as what is
spoken.*

ROSE
OFFNER

*I*f your henna paste is thinner in consistency, then small paintbrushes can be used to draw the designs. In Morocco, a hypodermic syringe without the needle is used as a tool to draw designs.

THE BOTTLE

An alternatively effective tool is a plastic Jacquard squeeze bottle which you can purchase. These applicator bottles are used in silk screening and batiking. The bottles can hold $1^{1}/2$ ozs. of paste and come with a choice of different sized removable metal tips. The #9 metal tip is fine for most designs.

An easy way to fill the bottle is to squeeze the henna paste from a cone into the bottle. While filling up the bottle with henna paste, tap the bottom against a hard surface periodically to release trapped air, then shake the henna paste to the tip. This can be a very good way to apply henna.

To apply henna from a bottle is really quite easy. Just squeeze and adjust the thickness of the line by the pressure you use from your fingertips on the sides of the bottle. Hold the bottle at an angle to the skin. As you use up the henna, shake it down towards the tip and fill up after using two-thirds of the henna, so you have a steady flow of paste.

To preserve the freshness of the paste, insert a straight pin into the metal tip. Clean the bottle after using it, washing out any henna. Left over henna might dry and clog the tip.

THE CONE

A cone is also one of the best and most popular ways to apply henna. The cone has the capability of holding a larger amount of henna paste which allows you to do many designs. You can adjust the size of the hole, so you can draw very intricate designs. Trimming the tip with scissors produces a larger hole. Be careful. Don't cut off too much. If you have rolled your cone tight on the tip, and use a gentle pressure when squeezing, you will have a very delicate line to do detailed work.

◄ *Indian henna artist preparing a bride for her wedding.*

MAKING A PLASTIC CONE

For centuries the sliver of wood or ivory were the only tools for henna artists. Just imagine. For our fast-paced world, sometimes this is just not effective.

Henna cones are similar to cake decorating cones. The difference is the henna cone has a smaller opening at the end. Pre-made cones can be purchased in stores that carry henna powder. But it is easy to make your own cone. All you need is a piece of medium thickness plastic or a plastic bag which can be purchased at the local grocery store. The size to buy is approximately 11" x 11" which will give you two pieces of plastic to roll two cones.

3. With one hand, hold one corner of the plastic square between your thumb and forefingers.

4. On that same side of the plastic square, with your other hand, place and hold your finger firmly on the other corner.

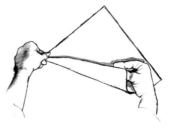

5. Now with your first hand, fold over the plastic and roll, while keeping your other finger firmly at the corner.

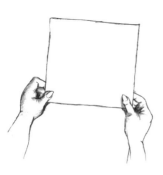

1. First cut along all four edges of the plastic bag cutting off 1/2 inch to remove the seams from the bag. You will then have 2 pieces of plastic.

2. Tear off 4 pieces of tape, each one inch long, to be used in step 7.

6. Hold the open end with your thumb and fore finger to maintain a shape, and roll by turning your wrist until you have a cone shape.

7. Hold the pointed end of the cone, and with the other hand place 2 strips of tape in the inside of the cone along the plastic seam, place a strip of tape along the seam on the outside of the cone, and one around the tip.

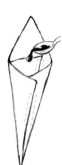

8. *Fill the cone with the henna paste with a rounded knife or a spoon. Each time you add henna paste squeeze the paste down towards the tip to remove air pockets.*

9. *Now, fold the top of the cone over several times. Tape down securely or wrap a rubber band around the cone to keep the paste in tightly. I like to wrap the entire cone with strong tape to make it a sturdier and more efficient tool.*

10. *Squeeze the cone. The paste should come out in a fine line. If it doesn't, very carefully trim the tip with manicure scissors. If the paste comes out in a line that is too thick, then the tip has been trimmed too much.*

▸ *Decorating with a henna cone.*

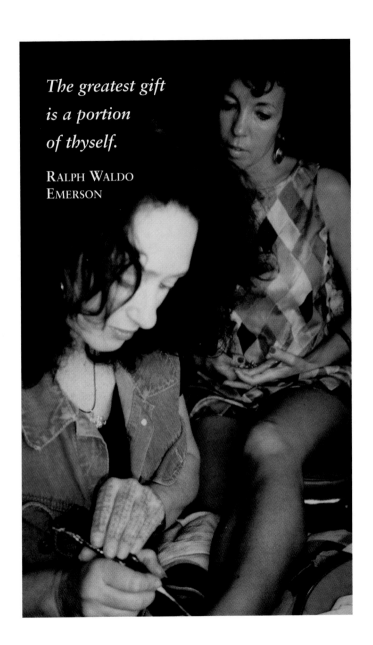

The greatest gift is a portion of thyself.

RALPH WALDO EMERSON

Making a Fast and Simple Cone

Here's an example of a cone that can be made quickly. Find a small plastic bag. Push the henna paste into one corner of the bag. Fold the rest of the bag around itself to form a cone shape. Tape securely and trim the tip. This type of cone is used to fill a plastic squeeze bottle, and by some to do design work, but I have found the cones made from a sheet of plastic more reliable and better for intricate work.

Using the Cone

Using the cone takes practice, so get yourself comfortable and try to relax your hands. It will make a big difference. Most of the time I hold the cone in two hands with the fingers of one hand near the tip. This is where I guide the henna to create the design and also where I use the most sensitive pressure to make either a very fine line or thicker line. My other hand is placed near the end of the cone and the pressure from these fingers gently pushes the henna towards the tip keeping a steady supply. At times I can use the cone with one hand nearest the tip.

I begin by squirting the henna out on a piece of tissue to test the consistency of the henna and to remove any air or dry henna that might be in the tip.

Then place the tip of the cone on the skin and let the henna form a line. Move the line along by moving the tip of the cone. This method is very good for detail work needing curves, circles and wavy lines. If you are going to draw a geometric design you can start by squeezing out the henna and then slowly lift up the tip of the cone enough so the henna will fall onto the skin. This technique is good for a design needing many long lines.

Lemon and Sugar

After you have finished applying your design, give it some time to settle in and dry. This takes from five to thirty minutes depending on the thickness of the henna. This is a crucial time for the design—while the henna is wet it is still very fragile. The slightest movement can disturb the design, and the paste can smear or move, and sharpness or detail can be compromised. So be sure the person who receives the design stays very still during this period or all your hard work is lost.

When the henna is sufficiently dry and before it starts to crack, dab a mixture of lemon and sugar onto the design. This is a very important part of the henna design procedure. The lemon and sugar mixture acts as a mordant, encouraging the henna to stain even darker, and the sugar makes the solution sticky, which keeps the henna on the skin for many hours.

Every henna artist has a favorite lemon-sugar combination. A good formula is two parts lemon juice to one part sugar. I sometimes mix an extra sticky solution of one part lemon juice to one part sugar. The added sugar ensures the henna will stay securely on the skin. Fresh squeezed lemon juice is best, but pre-squeezed juice will suffice. If you use fresh squeezed juice, be sure to strain it to catch all the seeds and pulp which you will discard. Stir the mixture until the sugar dissolves completely and don't worry about exact measurements.

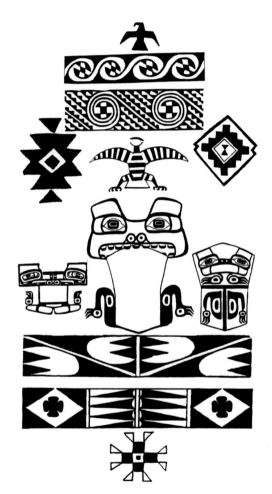

NORTH AMERICAN INDIAN

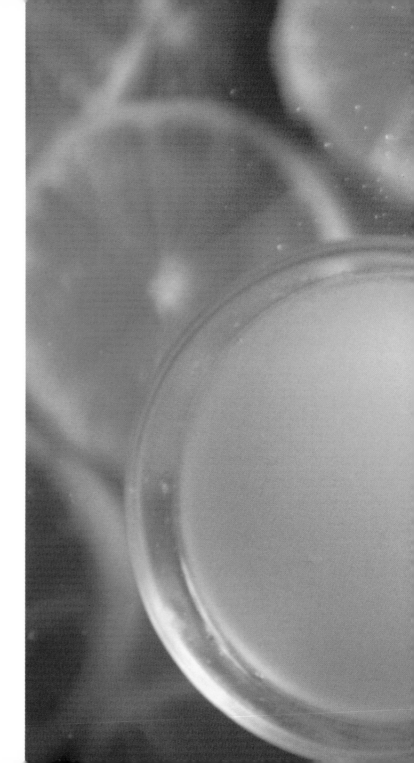

Applying the lemon and sugar to the design twice is a good idea. Use a cotton ball made of 100% cotton or a Q-tip and lightly dab the design when it is dry. Dab carefully so that the henna does not lift up. If the lemon-sugar mixture starts to drip, wipe it away quickly or you will have a drip line as part of your design. Applying the lemon and sugar twice is a good idea if the henna is thick. Wait until the first coat is dry and the henna begins to look crusty, then apply a second coat. This is when the henna is most fragile, so be very gentle.

When you are creating a large design, and you notice the first part of the design beginning to dry, you might want to stop and dab lemon and sugar on the dry part of the design. Continue designing and apply the lemon-sugar mixture to the rest of the design in sections.

▸ *The lemon and sugar solution.*

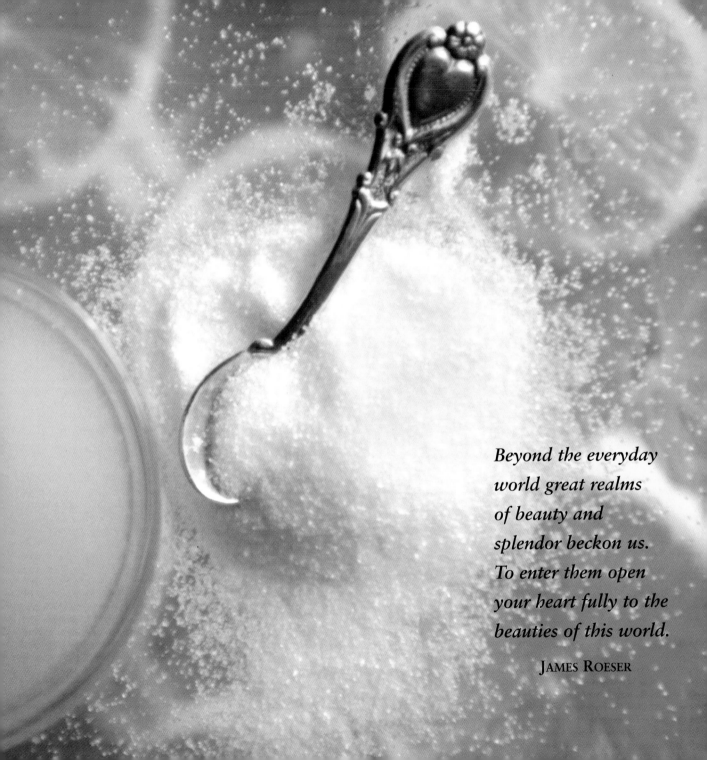

Beyond the everyday
world great realms
of beauty and
splendor beckon us.
To enter them open
your heart fully to the
beauties of this world.

JAMES ROESER

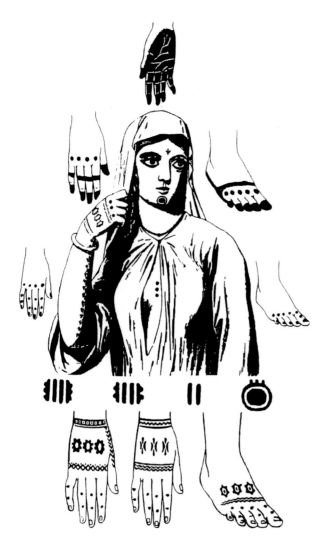

EGYPT

FOR A DEEPER DESIGN

Our skin temperature has a big influence on how strong the henna will stain. If at all possible, warming the skin after you have completed the design will, in most cases, make a difference. Warming the skin will open the pores so the design can stain more deeply. The henna will still stain in its lovely hues without this step, but for a little more depth in color, and a few extra days added to the life of the design, it is worth the effort.

There are several ways this can be accomplished. One is to hold the design over a candle or a lamp (heat lamps work great) to warm it up. You can also hold it over a hot pan filled with smoldering cloves. If this is convenient, or if you want to do what our henna ancestors have done, you can hold your design over the heat of a sultry evening fire.

PROTECTING AND ENHANCING THE DESIGN

If enough lemon and sugar have been applied to the design, the paste will have a shiny glazed surface. The design is pretty strong at this point and will survive the next twelve hours with little cracking off. Wrapping cotton, tissues, toilet paper or socks onto the design can further protect it. Keep your design out of water for 12 hours and don't use soap for 24 hours. Some also recommend keeping the design away from strong sunlight, which can inhibit the dying process of the henna.

The henna artists of Hawaii have found a way to lengthen the life of the henna design. They coat the henna design with mustard paste and a salad oil. They then wrap the design in plastic overnight. In Morocco, some artists have coated the henna paste with vinegar and garlic to get the same results.

REMOVING THE PASTE

When the time has come to remove the paste (6-12 hours after application) soak a cotton ball with a little almond, olive or mustard oil and massage it into the henna paste. Remove the paste entirely from the skin. Remember, no water or soap. Wait between one to three days for your design to secretly turn darker. Then you, and whomever you come in contact with, will enjoy the pleasures of henna designs.

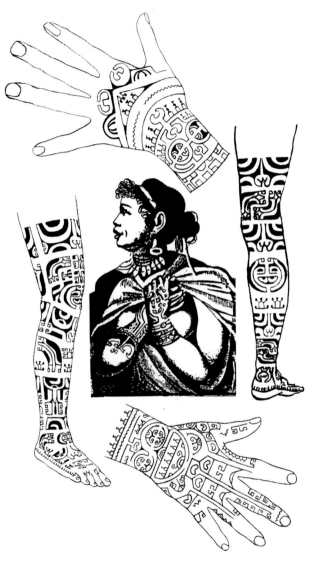

MAORI

A good place to start is with a stencil which is easy to use. I chose the stencils in this kit after much research and selected traditional designs from a variety of cultures. Some I have incorporated with my own patterns. I encourage you to enjoy henna with one of these patterns. They show you what is possible. Please experiment and modify them as you will. They are fast and easy to use. No experience is necessary. They are fun to use with friends so invite a few over for a stencil party. They are for your ease and pleasure.

The stencils are made from hypoallergenic material so it would be unlikely anyone would have an allergic reaction. If you have sensitive skin it is best to test the stencil on your skin before you apply henna paste.

1. Choose a good place for your design. For example, the long band designs can be placed on the wrist, the upper arm and the ankle. Circular or single design patterns can be placed on the top or bottom of the hand. The forearm, leg, navel, shoulder or back are also good places.

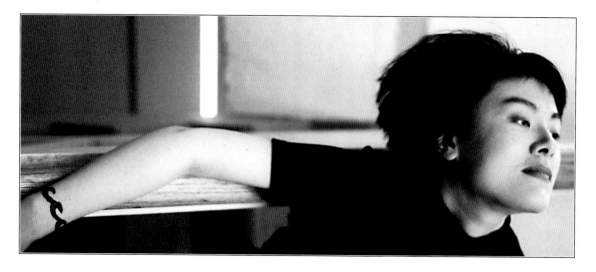

2. Hold the stencil in one hand and with the other hand pull the backing away from the adhesive side. Some stencil designs have several sections that need to be peeled off one at a time. This can be done before the backing is peeled off or on the skin after the stencil is put on.

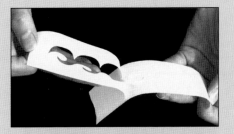

3. Now that you have opened the stencil, place the side with the adhesive on the area of the body you have chosen for your design. With your finger, press and pat all edges of the stencil firmly against the skin. This is to insure henna paste will not seep under the stencil.

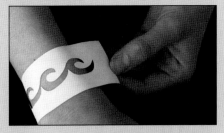

4. Apply the henna paste on the design area (a medium coat) and make sure you have covered the skin completely. You can use henna paste mixed from scratch or pre-mixed henna paste from the tube. Leave on for seven minutes.

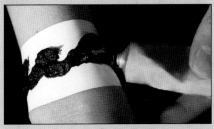

5. After seven minutes, slowly pull off. If needed, touch up the henna in the design with a toothpick. If you want to reuse the stencil, lightly place it on the stencil backing for later.

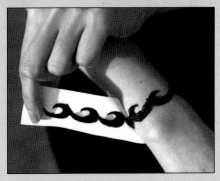

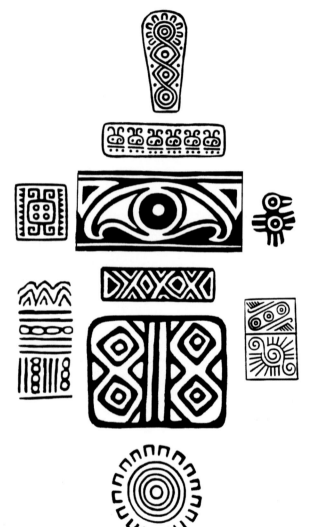

MAYAN

Remember when you were a child and you would draw freely without inhibition? The end result was not as important as the spontaneity and pleasure of creating. It didn't matter if anyone liked it or not. What mattered was your own delight in the doing. The henna experience is like that. Go back in time, relax and pretend you are a child. Somewhere inside you that child is alive and well. Let go of your judging self which has the doubts and misgivings. Be the henna artist you are. This is the best part.

In this section I will guide you step by step through the basics of henna application. Henna designing is very similar to drawing. If you are intimidated, begin by tracing a design on a piece of paper with a pencil. When you have chosen a design that feels right, you may wish to use some henna and practice on a piece of paper first to get comfortable. Or start right on the skin once you have chosen the right place to put it.

I have included simple drawing exercises on page 117 to help familiarize you with drawing some basic henna designs. Begin by practicing straight lines, curved lines, swirls and circles. Then build a design by adding several exercises together. Don't be timid. Experiment. It is temporary after all!

Beginning Geometric Design

A good design to start out with is this Mayan inspired geometric motif. This design is very attractive and easy to do. Don't be fooled. The simple designs can be just as beautiful and powerful as the more complicated ones, and they take less time to apply. For example, I placed this geometric design on the top of the hand but other areas of the body would also work, such as the palm of the hand and the top of the foot.

1. Locate the area where you want the design to be. Find the center of the design. Make a small dot.

2. Put 4 dots in the north, south, east and west corners.

3. Enlarge the middle dot and draw a circle around it.

4. Connect the outside dots with 4 straight lines to make a diamond shape.

5. Make 4 more dots a little distance away from each corner of the diamond shape.

6. Again connect the outside dots with straight lines.

7. Go back to the top corner. Apply a dot and go around the perimeter with dots about 1/4 inch apart.

8. Wait until it has dried and dab with lemon and sugar.

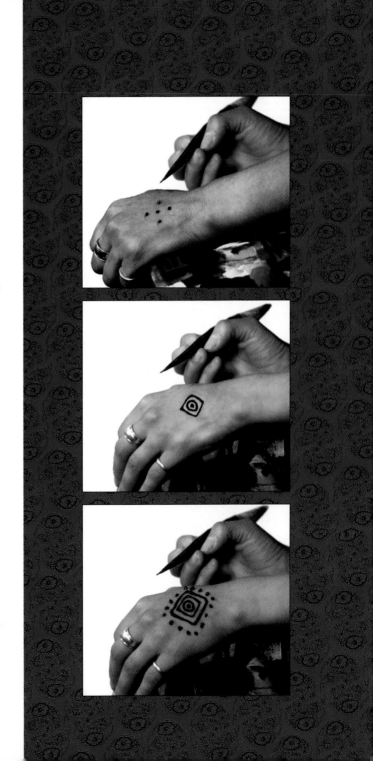

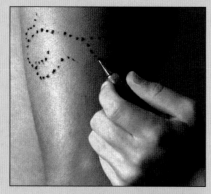

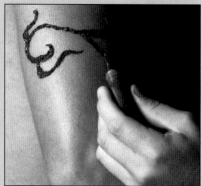

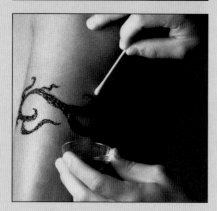

STEPS FOR A NEW TRIBAL DESIGN

There are many choices for the placement of designs. For example, a long new tribal design can be placed in different spots on the upper arm or on the ankle. A smaller band design would be great for the wrist. Don't limit yourself. Be adventurous and try different designs (look on page 120 for a selection). This design I have chosen is placed on the upper arm. Give it a try!

1. To begin, map in the design by putting little dots on the arm. This will help you keep the design straight.

2. Fill in the preliminary outline with henna paste.

3. Dab with lemon and sugar when the design is dry.

As you practice henna designing, you will create your own style and preferences. Positioning yourself and the person getting the design becomes a personal choice. Decide what is most comfortable for you. On page 119 I offer a offer a few suggestions that have worked for me. .

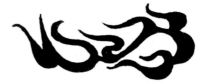

A variation of the design shown in the photos

BASIC FREE HAND EXERCISES

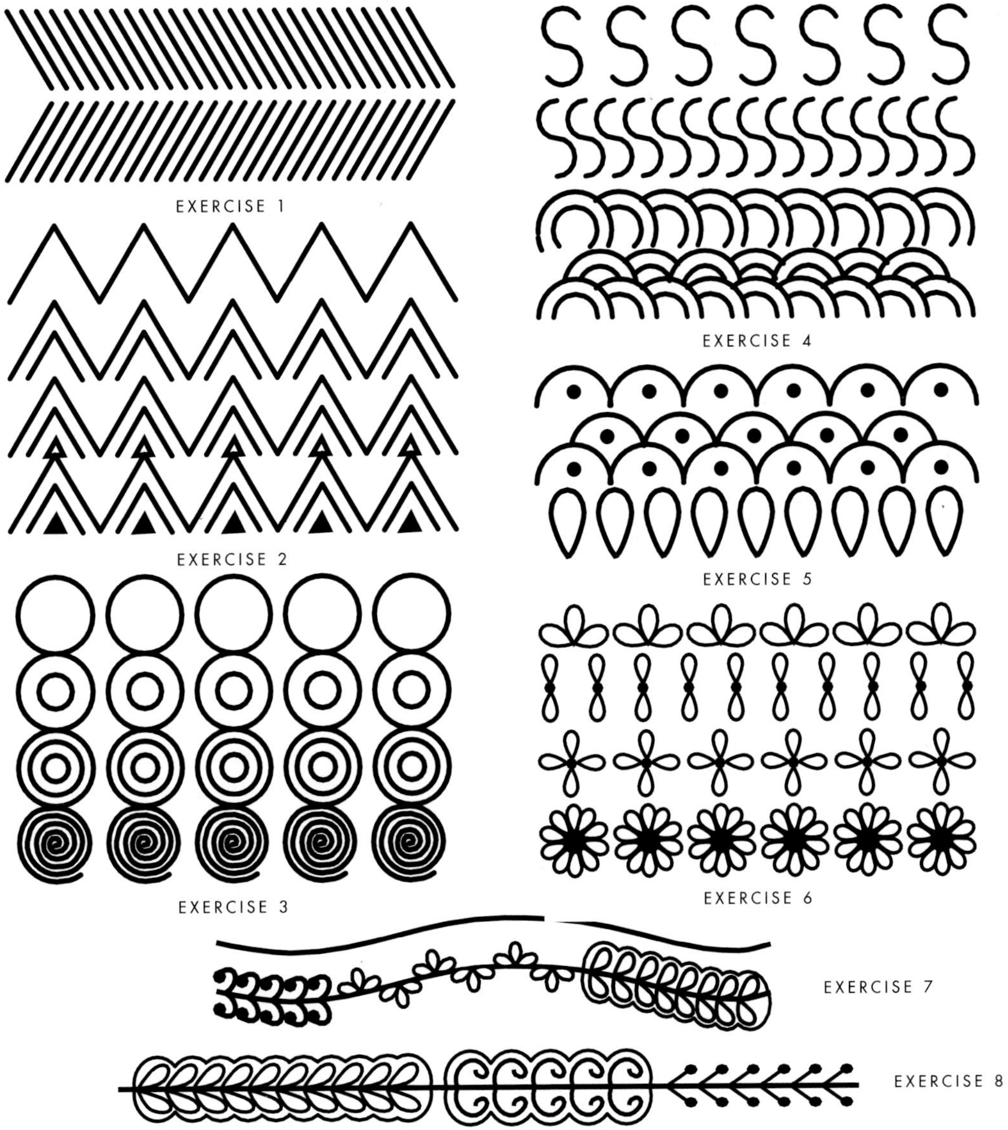

EXERCISE 1

EXERCISE 2

EXERCISE 3

EXERCISE 4

EXERCISE 5

EXERCISE 6

EXERCISE 7

EXERCISE 8

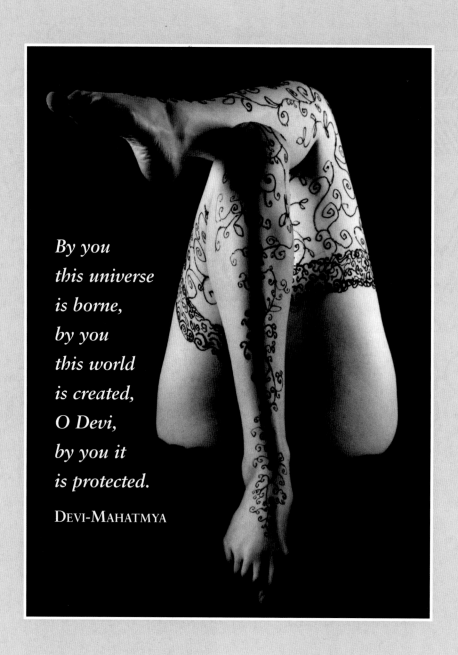

By you
this universe
is borne,
by you
this world
is created,
O Devi,
by you it
is protected.

DEVI-MAHATMYA

HANDS

If you are decorating just the tops of the hands, it is very easy. Simply place hands flat and decorate one at a time. If you are decorating both sides of the hands, here is the procedure I found works the best. Decorate one palm first. Wait until the paste dries. Carefully dab it with lemon and sugar before moving on. Design the top of the other hand next, then the other palm. Finally, decorate the top of the remaining hand. Arrange the arms and hands into a comfortable position, propping with pillows which you have covered with tissue to protect from staining. The hands can be braced by resting the fingertips against a table if they are not covered with paste. If you want to cover the fingertips, apply the paste last to them after all other designing. Stains on the fingertips and palms will be the deepest color. Stains on the fingernails and toenails will last several months.

ARMS

Bands and long thin designs are good choices for the arm. Bend the arm and place the elbow on a pillow. Apply small dots around the arm to ensure a straight line. (A very light yellow washable felt pen can also be used to draw out the design beforehand.) If the person is particularly muscular, it is better to have the arm hang straight down when the design is applied. This is because sometimes the surface of the arm will change shape when it is bent, and the design could then look crooked when the arm is straightened.

WRISTS

There are many choices for bracelet designs. Any of the border or band designs are very inspirational. Hold the arm up bent at the elbow and start designing the first side of the wrist. Then lower the arm and design the other side.

FEET

Feet are always spectacular to decorate. If the bottoms of the feet are part of the design, decorate them last. Before you begin, be aware that some people have very sensitive feet. If they are ticklish it will add a whole new dimension to the experience.

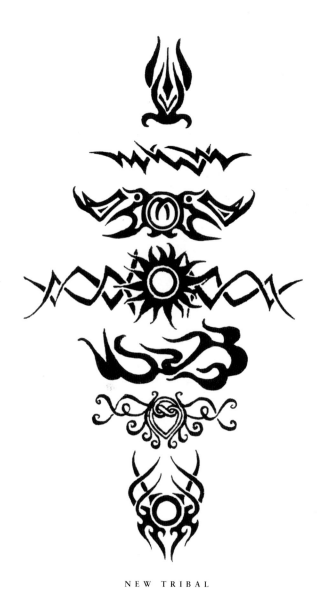

Start by decorating the tops of the feet. Move up towards the ankle. You can prop the feet in your lap or against the edge of a chair. To design up the ankle, have the person stand or lower the leg. You can prop it on a pillow. Remember, do not bend the ankle while the paste is wet or the design will smear. Sometimes at this point, it is best to sit on the floor to finish the design. But keep yourself comfortable. No strained backs or necks, please!

ANKLE

I find if the person stands with the foot flat on a chair or on the floor, I get the best results. Map the design with dots. Then apply the henna to the front side of the ankle. When it is complete, apply the henna to the back of the ankle and finish that portion of the design.

BACKS AND SHOULDERS

The best position for applying the back design is to have the person straddle a chair. This is very comfortable. Be careful as it is easy to fall asleep. I suggest drawing out the design on a piece of paper first to make sure the design follows the contour of the body. You might have to add or subtract a little for the design to fit. Remember not to lean against anything for a few hours or the design will be disturbed. It is well worth the extra effort.

MIDRIFF AND STOMACH

There are several ways to decorate these areas. The person can lie down, sit in a reclining position, or stand up. Smaller designs will work in the lying down position but you must draw between breaths. Each time the person breathes this area of the body will lift and the design will move or crack. It's not fair to ask them to hold their breath for 20 minutes, so take your time! Patch up the design if need be and give a hand when it's time to get up.

The larger designs work best if applied while the person is standing up or sitting in a reclining position. This is because this area of the body can shift a little when a person is upright. If a large design is applied while the person is lying down, when they get up the design can look irregular. The person should lean against something, take breaks, enjoy and in the spirit of henna notice the layers of life's tensions and stresses roll off. This is the magic of the art of henna.

VICTORIAN

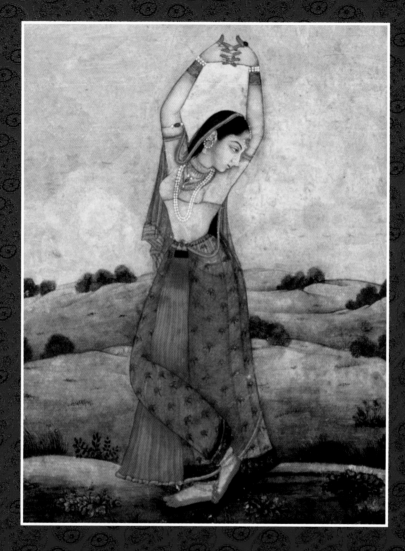

Where love reigns the impossible
may be obtained.

INDIAN PROVERB

These designs can be very intimidating because they look so complex and difficult. However, they can become very simple if planned and applied in sections. Most of the time the design has several main areas: the fingers, the central part of the design, and the upper part of the design near the wrist. Start with the central part. Next apply the henna to the fingers, then the wrist area and finish by filling in the rest of the design. Sometimes the design has an actual line or lines outlining these areas. It can help to henna in the main outlines that cordon off these sections first. Filling in these areas one at a time will make it less complicated. Apply the paste in such a fashion, usually away from yourself, to insure your hand will not smear or smudge the already hennaed areas.

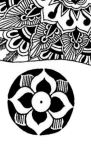

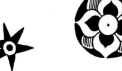

◄ *"Mughal Dancer," 18th Century. Mughal Indian miniature painting showing hennaed hands and feet.*

INDIA

THE IMPORTANCE OF HENNA

My personal experience of henna on my own body, and as I have applied it to others, has revealed that a certain magic occurs—the magic of connection. Somehow, as we sit quietly and take time out of our fast-paced, frenzied lives to be touched and adorned, we remember our roots. We connect to each other, to our past and deeply within to ourselves. I can explain it in no other way. We humans have always longed for rituals that directly connect us to spirit. We are longing for this in our hectic and disjointed modern culture. To participate in henna takes us right back to our ancestors. The ancient symbols and designs in henna decoration cut through all boundaries of time and space.

Over the centuries, women would teach the art of henna and pass its beautiful designs and henna recipes on to each other. As these women would apply the designs they would chat, tell stories and create small traditions. A way of living was created from one generation to another. We join this long tradition when we decide to participate in henna. Universally, henna transcends all social categories, all classes, all ages, all religions, all politics. It deals with the hidden, the mysterious, the revealed. It is the gate from culture to nature and from nature back to culture. It brings love, happiness, protection, beauty, connection and joy.

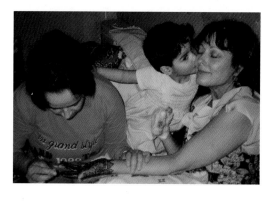

◄ *Moroccan henna artist applying henna.*
▸ *A Mauritius Island bride beautifully decorated with henna.*

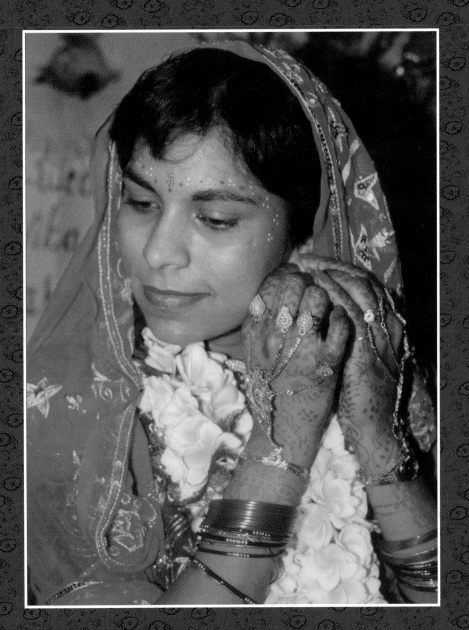

*Oh my Queen,
Queen of
the Universe,
the Queen who
encompasses
the universe,
may your beloved
enjoy long days
at your side.*

FROM A
SUMERIAN TEXT

BIBLIOGRAPHY

BOOKS

Achterberg, Jeanne. *Woman as Healer.* Boston: Shambala, 1991.

Agrawal, Pushpa, *Evergreen Mehandi Designs.* Ahmadabad: Navaneet Publications Limited.

Allende, Isabel. *Aphrodite: A Memoir of the Senses.* New York: Harper Collins, 1998.

Bhavnani, Enakshi. *Decorative Designs and Craftmanship of India.* Bombay: Russi Jal Taraporevala, 1969.

Corson, Richard. *Fashions in Makeup from Ancient to Modern Times.* London: Peter Owen Limited, 1972.

Croutier, Alev Lytle. *Taking the Waters, Spirit, Art, Sensuality.* New York: Abbeville Press, 1992.

Grafton, Carol Belanger. *Treasury of Japanese Designs and Motifs for Artists and Craftsmen.* New York: Dover Publications, Inc., 1983.

Guiliani, Bob. *Animal Illustrations.* New York: Dover Publications, Inc., 1988.

Kapchan, Deborah and Young, K., ed. *Bodylove.* Knoxville: University of Tennessee Press, 1993.

Kinsley, David. *Hindu Goddesses.* Delhi: The Regents of the University of California, 1987.

Kirtikar, Lt. Colonel K.R. *Indian Medicinal Plants.* Dehradun: International Book Dist.

Krakow, Amy. *Tattoo Book.* New York: Warner Books, Inc., 1994.

Lane, Edward William. *Manners and Customs of the Egyptians.* London: J.M. Dent & Sons Ltd., 1860.

Lsun, Ming-Ju. *Oriental Floral Designs and Motifs for Artists, Needleworkers and Craftspeople.* New York: Dover Publications, Inc., 1985.

Lucas, A. and Harris, J.R. *Ancient Egyptian Materials and Industries.* London: Histories & Mysteries of Man Ltd., 1989.

Meader, Jonathan. *In Praise of Women.* Berkeley: Celestial Arts, 1997.

Miller, Jean-Chris. *The Body Art Book.* New York: The Berkeley Publishing Group, 1997.

Pearce, Mallory. *Ready To Use Celtic Designs.* New York: Dover Publications, Inc., 1995.

Phoenix and Arabeth. *Henna (Mehndi) Bodyart Handbook: Complete How-To Guide.* Phoenix and Arabeth, 1997.

Poucher, William A. *Perfumes, Cosmetics and Soaps: Vols. 1 and 2.* New York: D. Van Nostrand Company, Inc., 1942.

Robley, Major-General. *Moko or Maori Tattooing.* London: Chapman Hall Ltd., 1896.

Sangl, Harry. *The Blue Privilege: The Last Tattooed Maori Women.* Auckland: Richards Publishers in association with W. Collins, 1980.

Searight, Susan. *The Use and Function of Tattooing on Moroccan Women.* New Haven: HRA Flex Books, MW1-001 Ethnography Series, 1984.

Smedt, Marc de. *The Kama-Sutra Erotic Figures in Indian Art.* New York: Crescent Books, 1980.

Williams, Geoffrey. *African Designs.* New York: Dover Publications, Inc., 1971.

Wilson, Eva. *North American Indian Designs.* New York: Dover Publications, Inc., 1987.

ARTICLES

Encyclopedia Brittanica. Vol. XIII pp. 271. New York: Encyclopeaedia Brittanica, Inc., 1911.

Holland, Barbara. *"Cleopatra: What Kind of a Woman Was She, Anyway?"* , Smithsonian, Feb., 1997, Vol. 27 Issue 11 p. 56.

Kapchan, Deborah and Young, K., ed.. *"Moroccan Women's Body Signs"*, Bodylove. Knoxville: University of Tennessee Press,1993.

Messina, Maria. *"Henna Party: An Orange-Red Cosmetic Raises Moroccan Women's Spirits,"* Natural History, 1988, Vol. 97 (9).

World Book Encyclopedia, Vol. 1 p. 733. Chicago: The World Book Encyclopedia, 1984.

World Book Encyclopedia, Vol. 4 p. 512. Chicago: The World Book Encyclopedia, 1984.

PERMISSIONS

Poem p. 4 used by permission of Rebecca Boyd. Quotation p. 18 used by permission of Mynya Giballawinsky. Quotation p. 22 used by permission of Barbara Demeter. Song/poem p. 29 used by permission of Roo Cantada. Painting p. 30 "Spirit of India," artist unknown; courtesy of Barbara Sansone. Poem p. 44 from *He Smiled to Himself*, Berkeley: Shakti Press, © 1990 by Steve Sanfield; used by permission of Steve Sanfield. "North American Indian Courtship Song" on p. 61 from *American Indian Poetry* by Geoge W. Cronyn, ed. Copyright © 1918 and renewed 1962 by George W. Cronyn. Reprinted by permission of Ballantine Books, a Division of Random House Inc. Quotation p. 72 used by permission of Kachinas Kutenae. Poem p. 86 from *Holy Uncertainty, collection #9*, by Steve Sanfield; used by permission of Steve Sanfield. Quotation p. 102 from *Journal to Intimacy*, by Rose Offner, Berkeley: Celestial Arts, © 1997; used by permission of Rose Offner. Illustrations pp. 104–105 by Leo Foster. Quotation p. 109 used by permission of James Roeser. Painting p. 122 courtesy of the Asian Art Museum of San Francisco. Excerpts on pp. 25, 49, and 62 are from the poem "I am the Goddess of Fertility" by Isabel Allende are reprinted from *In the Praise of Women*, Jonathan Meader, ed., Berkeley: Celestial Arts, copyright © 1997; used by permission of Isabel Allende.

PHOTOGRAPHY AND MODEL CREDITS

Note: Henna artist for all photographs is Pamela Nichols unless otherwise noted.

GALE BEASLEY
p.62, model: Julianne K. Stahl

SOPHIA BOWART
p.68, model: Brian Lilla, p.64, model: Marc Clausen

SAJAN BOYJOO
p.2, model: Kavita Welsh, henna artist: Soudevi Boyjoo p.125, model: Kavita Welsh

JAY DANIEL
p.25, model: Maria Lisa Buehl, p.44, model: Gail Weissman

KATHRYN DEDMEN
p.105, model: Pamela Nichols / Marjorie Stark

MICHAEL FAHEY
p.8, model: Maria Lisa Burke

GEORGE W. GERHARD
p.124, model: unknown / unknown, Kathleen Gerhard,
henna artist: unknown Moroccan artist

AARON LAUER
p.12 & p.78, model: Rosemary Todd-Sanchez,

MING LOUIE
p.14 & p.15, model: Jenna Louie, p.70 & p.71, model: Norma Tringali

PAMELA NICHOLS
p.22, model: Kayetana Klinghoffer

PRISCILLA PATEY
p.85, model: John James Bramell, henna artist: Priscilla Patey

BARBARA SANSONE
p.67, model: Jesse Nichols

ROBERT STEWART
p.72, model: MacKenzie Fotsch/April'the cat'
p.81, model: Sina Tyrell, p.76–77, model: Pam Nichols / Mandala Grace Kowal
p.20–21, model: Luciana L Foster, p.7 & p.10–11, model: Angela Weasa
p.4 & p.61, model: Aja Jayme-Wolf, p.26 & p.35, model: Kayetana Klinghoffer

PASCALE TREICHLER
Cover, p.50, model: Oceana Rain Stuart, p.74 & p.75, model: Shelby French,
p.39, model: Rosemary Todd-Sanchez, p. 18, 82, 86, 92, 93

JEANETTE VONIER
p.56, model: Jasmine Rose Nichols, p.49, model: Erin McConnel
p.43, model: Maria Lisa Burke, p.118, model: Victoria Howell

SVEN WIEDERHOLT
p.40, model: Joy Jones, p.96, model: Sanaz Kafayi, p.16, model: Luciana L. Foster,
p.29, model: Dea Fredrick, p.112–113 (series of 3 photos), model: Lulu Kwok

JONATHAN R. ZINSMEYER
p.115, model: Roo Cantada (series of 3 photos)
p.116, model: Justin Barr/ Brendon Barr (series of 3 photos),
p.540, model: Brendon Barr, p.108–109

PHOTOGRAPHER UNKNOWN
p.32, 38, 102, model: Anu Bhatia, henna artist: unknown
p.36, model: Bhatia family, henna artist: unknown

ACKNOWLEDGMENTS

My greatest appreciaton goes to henna artists throughout time. The joy recieved from henna designs has nurtured this beautiful art form for centuries and will for centuries to come.

For those who worked on this project I am greatly appreciative.

Thank you David Hinds of Celestial Arts for your eternal belief in me; Peter Beren my publishing consultant for your innovative ideas; to Bruce Wilson of Healthy Planet for your enthusiasm and strength, and to Scott Foster for making the mark.

Thanks to the people at Ten Speed Press: Phil Wood, Jo Ann Deck, Kirsty Melville, and Veronica Randall.

Thank you to Grace Brumett for your creative editing and support while burning those midnight oils; Leslie Waltzer for your perpetual energy and beautiful design; and to Janet Vail for your artful steadiness with the challenges of production.

Thanks to John West, Jim Battle, Rodney Grisso, Cindy Peer, Micah Johnson, Daniel Turbeville, Evan McKay, Jon Gerhard, Rod Pena, Sandy Brim, Sandra Maher, and to Anu Bhatia, your friends and your family for your historical research on the art of henna in India.

Many thanks to Meg McDonnell, Steve Turner, Peter Landis, the Rosicrucian Museum, the Indian Counsel of San Francisco, the Asian Art Mueseum of San Francisco, the Mill Valley library, the Anthropological Library at U.C. Berkeley, and all the photograhers and models who gave generously of their time.

Special thanks to my family and friends for their incredible love & support.

My father for your encouragement; my daughters Oceana, Jasmine and Mandala for your time, faith and enthusiasm in sharing my passion, my sons-in-law Edmundo Sarti, John Wondergem and Edward Balinski for your spirit; my brother Bob Nichols for supporting me when I needed it, my sister Linda Fotsch for your million-dollar advice, and to Pearlann Adrians, Johnny Strauss, Penny Quintner, and the Barr family.

Rebecca Boyd for you prophetic and angelic words of wisdom, Jeanne Schacker for our life-long, caring friendship; to Lama Jinpa Zangpo for your translations and guidance; to Norma Tringali for empowering my being.

Thank you to Bill Bullock for your powerful support and uncanny advice, to Warren Williams for being there, to Maggie McCoy and Richard Bittner for your support and first draft proofreading.

Special thanks to Jonathan Meader for your kindness; and to Rose Offner, Lois Anderson, Karena Oberman, Persia Matine, Duncan Fitzgerald, James Roeser, Debra Cooper, Barbara Summers, Raymond Himmel, Pamela Abramson-Levine, Dr. Barbara Custer, Ellen Cutler, Gregory Purnell, and Dr. Rafael Rettner.